SELLING HOPE BY THE POUND

You followed the rules, ate the RyKrisp, and, for a time, lost the weight. Your metabolism slowed, your weight rose, and there you were back where you started or worse. After years, you have discovered that, in the long run, dieting actually makes you *gain* weight. But you assume that's your fault. The diets work; you fail.

Unfortunately, there is a huge industry ready and waiting to take advantage of this confusion. The industry makes its services seem so accessible and its solutions so reasonable that hundreds of thousands of people understandably invest their time and money in them.

And it's a waste.

IF YOU'VE NEVER BEEN ON A COMMERCIAL DIET PROGRAM, DON'T START NOW.

IF YOU'VE BEEN ON SEVERAL PROGRAMS (AND YOU WEIGH MORE THAN WHEN YOU STARTED), STOP THE PROCESS NOW.

DIANE EPSTEIN is a psychologist with more than 20 years' experience in weight-control counseling and a former counselor to one of the major diet centers. **KATHLEEN THOMPSON** is coauthor of the classic *Against Rape*.

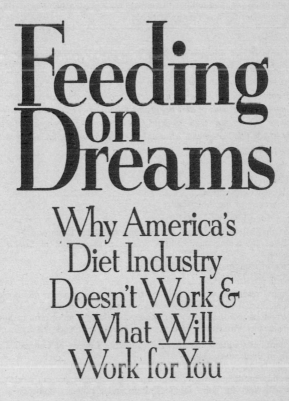

Feeding on Dreams

Why America's Diet Industry Doesn't Work & What Will Work for You

Diane Epstein & Kathleen Thompson

AVON BOOKS 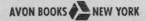 NEW YORK

In this book, we sometimes criticize specific practices engaged in by particular diet programs, which we have identified by name. By our criticisms, we do not mean to imply that every office of the identified programs engages in the practices described. Elsewhere, we express certain general criticisms of diet programs without referring to any program by name. We do not mean to imply that all of these general criticisms apply to each diet program, although they do reflect significant problems in the industry.

AVON BOOKS
A division of
The Hearst Corporation
1350 Avenue of the Americas
New York, New York 10019

Copyright © 1994 by Diane Epstein and Kathleen Thompson
Published by arrangement with Scribner's, an imprint of Simon and Schuster
Library of Congress Catalog Card Number: 93-33431
ISBN: 0-380-72521-5

The Scribner's edition contains the following Library of Congress Cataloging in Publication Data:
Epstein, Diane
    Feeding on dreams : why America's diet industry doesn't work—and what will work for you / Diane Epstein and Kathleen Thompson.
        p.   cm.
Includes bibliographical resources.
1. Reducing. 2. Reducing—United States. I. Thompson, Kathleen.
1946–   . II. Title.
RM222.2.E67 1994
613.2'5—dc20   93-33431
                                                                    CIP

First Avon Books Printing: March 1996

AVON TRADEMARK REG. U.S. PAT. OFF. AND IN OTHER COUNTRIES, MARCA REGISTRADA, HECHO EN U.S.A.

Printed in the U.S.A.

RA   10   9   8   7   6   5   4   3   2   1

To Troy Doetch, whose respect, trust, and healing have affected both our lives so profoundly that he actually made this book possible, and to Allen Askew, whose counseling philosophy served as an inspiration in Diane's life and her work.

Contents

Acknowledgments

WE WOULD LIKE to thank, for their help and encouragement, Geri Thoma, the staff of Sense and Nonsense, members of the Saturday morning workshop, Laura Dare, Pat Pakin, Phyllis Hirsch, Emily Calvo, Anita Young, Vicki Wolfson, Kathy O'Malley, Sara Thompson, Dian Barth, Michael Nowak, Terry Sullivan, Janne King, Anthony Lamberis, Beryl Heller, Albert Pinkert, Florence Pinkert, Frances Thompson, Les Thompson, Jr., and all of the people who agreed to share their stories with us.

Introduction

> *If American men are obsessed with money, American women are obsessed with weight. The men talk of gain, the women talk of loss, and I do not know which talk is more boring.*

MARYA MANNES

AS THIS BOOK is being written, there is a Jenny Craig commercial in which she compares dieting to having your hair done or going to the dentist. It's a particularly overt statement of something that has been part of the American consciousness for a long time.

Dieting is just a part of taking care of your appearance. Of course you do it over and over. It's an element of good grooming.

You don't even have to be above average in weight. "I had a beautiful figure," says Meryl, a diet program veteran, "but my mother brought home all this stuff to put my sister on a diet. She was ten, I was twelve. There was such a fuss over my sister, and lots of girls in eighth grade were on diets. So I did it. I thought it was terrific. I drank the diet pop and had the hard boiled eggs and grapefruit. It was easy. I've been dieting ever since."

For most of us, the first diet doesn't come quite that much out of the blue, but it's often close. If your top was a size eight and your bottom a size twelve—the American national average—you just decided one day to "take a little weight off" the lower half. It didn't seem like a particularly momentous decision. Not like getting your hair bleached or something.

> *A man has his clothes made to fit him;*
> *a woman makes herself fit her clothes.*

> EDGAR WATSON HOWE

And it seemed to make sense that you could become smaller. Everyone said it was simple; you take in fewer calories than you burn and you will lose weight. You could do that. You *did* do that. You followed the rules, ate the RyKrisp, and, for a time, lost the weight. It seemed that it ought to work that way. It still seems that it ought to work that way. However, as we'll explain later, it doesn't. As soon as you started dieting, your body started trying to protect itself against starvation. Your metabolism slowed, your weight rose, and there you were back where you started or worse. After that, another diet was the obvious solution.

That's all it takes—a couple of diets, a body that is working harder and harder to keep you from starving to death, and bingo! A weight problem for life.

The following is from a physical education textbook called *Movement Fundamentals,* by Janet Wessel. It was used in colleges when many baby boomers were in school.

> *A shapely figure calls for harmony of proportion. To be rightly proportioned, according to dress size, the waistline is 8 to 10 inches smaller than the bust circumference. The abdomen should measure from 1 ½ to 2 ½ inches smaller than the bust. The hips are usually 1 to 2 inches larger than the bust. Full hips measure 3 to 4 inches larger, while slim hips measure the same as the bust. Your calf should be*

4 to 5 inches larger than your ankle. Your thigh should be 10 to 13 inches larger than your ankle.

Pretty specific, huh? This was at the top of a page on which the student was to record her own measurements (taken by a partner) and, next to them, what the book called "proportional measurements." Part of the physical education course was training in "correcting" those proportions.

Today we know just how absurd this whole procedure was. But that eighteen-year-old who, at five foot six, weighed 114 pounds and wished to change her half-inch deviations from perfection, is now a forty-six-year-old with a lifelong history of diets.

And today's knowledge has changed only the *character* of the pressure for perfection. We no longer believe in our ability to manipulate the body's proportions quite that precisely without surgery. Now the pressure is simply to *reduce* them as much as possible, to alter them to fit today's fashion.

That pressure is the primary cause of most dieting. The problem is not trying to lose ten, fifteen, or twenty pounds. It is trying to lose weight that your body doesn't want to lose.

A study in the International Journal of Eating Disorders of 5,536 sorority women in the United States and Canada reported that 6.1 percent met the screening criteria for bulimia.

"Thunder thighs. It's what I call myself," says Randi, a Weight Watchers client who has been on and off that program for years. When she's smartly dressed in a long skirt and blazer, you wouldn't have a clue as to why she is so unhappy with her body. Her doctor claims that, like her mother, Randi is carrying an "excess" fifteen or twenty pounds. The doctor doesn't seem to notice that all her extra weight is in her very rounded hips and her large, muscular legs. Randi's waist is very small. Her shoulders and arms are beautiful. Even her belly is almost flat. In the area where fat can conceivably be dangerous—around the midriff—she has none. In addition to diets, Randi has tried every spot-reducing gimmick that comes on the market. She struggles to lose that fifteen pounds. Everyone says her face already looks drawn. But she still hates the way she looks in a pair of shorts.

And then there is the man we'll call Butch. He is in his middle thirties and played football in high school. By the time he graduated from college, he was battling the bulge. His solution to the problem is to go on a yearly diet. Every fall he loses twenty pounds. Over the rest of the year he gains them back. Only now he's gaining back more and finding it harder to lose. He doesn't seem to have the guilt that plagues so many women yo-yoers, probably because society doesn't disapprove so thoroughly of his shape. But he is worried about his health, and his jokes about his weight are getting strained.

It all comes back to that, again and again. You started dieting to lose weight. After years, you have discovered that, in the long run, dieting actually makes you *gain* weight. But you assume that's your fault. The diets work; you fail.

Lately you've been hearing a lot about diets not working. When you're at a party these days and someone says something negative about diets, you probably agree that diets are unhealthy and not very effective. But if you find people who still diet, you're more than ready to trade diet tips with them. You don't really believe that diets don't work. You've lost weight on every single one you've been on. And you've been on dozens.

Or maybe you haven't. You may be in your teens, deciding that the body you have gotten along with pretty well until now is not exactly what you want. You feel that you have just *got* to get rid of those thighs. Preferably before summer vacation. You *can't* show up at the lake looking like a beached whale.

Or maybe you're in your twenties, about to get married. You've never bothered much about your weight, but you'd really *love* to look thin and beautiful in your wedding dress. If you could only lose about twenty pounds, that special day would be perfect.

Perhaps you're hitting your late thirties or early forties and the slowdown is starting. *You* are slowing down and your metabolism is slowing down and the combination is putting inches onto your waist.

Or maybe you just quit smoking.

Thinking about weight may be just something that uses up energy and saps confidence you can't afford to lose. Or it may be something that consumes your every waking moment. Either way, we have news.

There is hope. You can significantly improve your situation. You can be happier, healthier, and, probably, thinner. You can get the problem under control and your life back in your own hands again. And if you're not yet trapped, the prognosis is really excellent.

There's been a lot of research into this problem, and things are finally starting to fall into place. We know better than ever what can be done and what needs to be done.

And yet, in spite of this progress, most people don't know what to think, don't know what to eat, and don't know where to turn. Some are frustrated and unhappy. Some are in constant pain and real danger.

Unfortunately, there is a huge industry ready and waiting to take advantage of this confusion. The industry makes its services seem so accessible and its solutions so reasonable that hundreds of thousands of people very understandably invest their time and money in them.

And it's a waste.

It would be bad enough if the investment were a waste only of time and money. But, for far too many people, what gets wasted is their determination to change, their confidence in their ability to have a different life, and their sense of self-worth. Such diet programs as Jenny Craig, Nutri/System, and Physicians Weight Loss have so much money and such good advertising agencies that they can make themselves very appealing. A great many of us have either signed on the dotted line or considered it. This most visible and attractive of options has to be put into perspective and, with any luck, put out of business.

So, although the second half of the book will tell you what you can do about your weight, we will begin by telling you what not to do and why. Simply stated, if you have never been on a commercial diet program, don't start now. If you have been on several programs (and you weigh more than when you started), stop the process now.

What gives us the confidence to make such an unequivocal statement?

Well, diet programs do not release—and insist that they do not keep—records of their successes and failures. (Optifast is the single exception, and their results were *not good.*) However, recent studies have indicated that four out of every five people who join a diet center program will not stay with the program long enough to lose *any* significant amount of weight. That's four out of five! *Eighty percent of the paying customers* go away with absolutely no satisfaction—only a feeling of personal failure because they didn't have the "willpower" to stick with it.

Again, studies indicate that only one out of ten of those who manage to lose even twenty-five pounds on a diet program will keep the weight off for as long as two years. That's only one in ten of the *one in five* who lost any weight at all.

To go further, one in fifty will keep it off for seven years. In other words, out of every two hundred and fifty people who enroll in a commercial weight loss program, *one* will have a longterm weight loss.

If, with our office copiers, we got a copy only once out of every two hundred and fifty times we tried, if AT&T managed to complete only one out of every two hundred and fifty phone calls, if only one of every two hundred and fifty photos taken actually produced a picture, there would be a consumer revolution.

> *1 out of 5 diet program clients loses any weight at all.*
> *1 out of 10 of those "successful" clients keeps the weight off for two years.*
> *1 out of 50 keeps the weight off for as long as seven years.*
> *In other words, 1 out of 250 will have a longterm weight loss.*
>
> *The rest, all 249 of them, will gain their weight back and, usually, more.*

And no diet program has ever been able to show results better than this.

Furthermore, gaining the weight back does not simply return you to your starting point. There is a great deal of evidence piling up that this repeated "lose and gain" pattern leaves you in a position that is physically and emotionally compromised.

It's true. At a time when the medical establishment is finally beginning to admit that "extra weight" is not usually a health problem, yo-yo dieting is under attack. Recent medical studies indicate that the health risks for people who regularly lose and gain significant amounts of weight are greater than for those who remain stable, even if significantly over the average weight. Articles in the *New England Journal of Medicine* and other sources indicate that losing and gaining even fifteen or twenty pounds periodically can cause stress to your heart muscle, in addition to an increase in your overall percentage of body fat.

In other words, repeated dieting increases your risk of heart disease *and* makes you fatter.

Our opinion, that diet programs create problems instead of solving problems, is based not only on all the recent books and articles indicting diet and the diet industry. We did more than gather all of the independent studies that reveal the diet programs to be similar in outcome and worthless. We conducted dozens of interviews with clients and diet program staff. (Many of the clients had been successful in losing weight; all of them had gained back the weight after the program.) Much of our book is based on personal observation of the diet industry at work, from the perspective of the counselor.

We talked to people from all of the major companies. The staff interviews followed a questionnaire. The client interviews were less formal. They included a few simple questions:

- Which diet programs have you tried?

- What motivated you to go on this particular program?

- How did the program work? (What was the process of signing up? What was the program's diet? What were the company services? What was required of you?)

- What were the results of your experience? (How long were you on the program? How did you like the diet? What did you think about the staff? Did you learn anything in the program? What was your weight loss or gain? Do you feel the program had any lasting impact?

- Would you go on this or another program again? Why?

The responses to these questions are scattered throughout the book in quotes and in client stories. They speak more emphatically of the program abuses than any set of statistics. They make a stronger argument against diet programs than we could possibly make by presenting the numbers and the failures.

Many of the responses we got from clients and staff went beyond the questionnaire or interview. Surprisingly, even some of the currently employed program staff were willing to speak candidly about their experiences (as long as their names were withheld.) Clients, of course, were more than happy to discuss all the details of their diet efforts.

In the second chapter, where we describe the diet programs, we have not ordered the programs or rated them in any way to imply good, bad, better, or worse. Although some programs are more unrealistic or ridiculous than others, that sort of evaluation would be deceptive because, very simply, *none of them work and all of them are potentially harmful.* We'll prove that to you.

One of us—Diane Epstein—has spent twenty years counseling people with weight problems and eating disorders, and many of her individual clients and the members of her workshops have contributed their experiences to this book. Both of us have spent most of our lives dealing with these issues personally. This book was inspired by Diane's experiences while serving on the staff of a major diet center chain.

At first, we planned to devote this entire book to exposing the deceptive practices of those centers. But, as we worked on the book and talked to people about it, we discovered that outrage would carry us only so far. We couldn't condemn the diet industry without offering alternatives, especially when those alternatives were so effective. Indeed, offering alternatives is exactly what Diane ended up doing while still working for that diet center chain. She began closing the door and being honest to the clients who came to her for counseling, just as she was honest with the clients in her own individual counseling practice.

She didn't have any other choice.

Diane found that she was unable to tell a bulimic woman that she couldn't sign up without also telling her that she could find help in other ways. She couldn't let a mother of three spend every penny she could squeeze from her household budget on foods that were higher in fat and lower in nutrition than the food she was serving her family without pointing out that there were other options.

So, here's what we know.

You have to start where you are in this whole dieting/

weight/eating/moving business. The diet programs make you feel that not only do you have the Wrong Body, you also have the wrong tastes, cravings, and enjoyments. According to them, some of the greatest joys of your life— french fries, fudge brownies, cream sauce—are just cheap thrills.

> *A study of three thousand people that was reported in the British Medical Journal revealed that the fattest subjects ate the least and the thinnest ate the most.*

Well, don't believe them for a minute. Life offers few sensual pleasures greater than chocolate. You'd have to be crazy to give it up. What you like to eat is as much a part of who you are as what you like to read, wear, or do on your vacation. No matter what the scale says, you are entitled to food that you choose, food that satisfies you and gives you pleasure. And we're going to show you how to get back to that.

You also don't have to start jogging and doing step aerobics in the morning. Taken slowly and incorporated gradually into your lifestyle, exercise can be one of life's great pleasures, as well as the surest way to modify your shape. But what you can handle right off may be nothing more than walking in place in front of your television for five minutes. If you start there, you may eventually end up hiking the Appalachian Trail. But if you don't start there, if you push yourself even a little too hard, you'll end up back on the couch. We're going to help you deal with exercise resistance, boredom, pain, sweat, and all the other things that keep you sitting on your setpoint (more on that later).

What's more, how you eat and how you move are only a part of the answer. In some cases, a very small part.

If you were to sit down with an individual weight control counselor, the two of you would talk about your history and your feelings, when weight became an issue for you and what you've done about it. You could work out together where you should start and what's most important and what kind of help you need. We're going to try to come as close to that as we can. We won't just tell you things. We'll ask you. And your answers will be as important as anything else in this book. Fill out the questionnaires. Do the exercises. This isn't a novel.

It also isn't your average self-improvement book. For one thing, we're going to operate on the assumption that you have a pretty good "self," all things considered, and what needs to be improved is what's happening to it.

Second, there's a certain feeling you get when reading that sort of book, a feeling that the authors are talking to you and you alone, and that everything they say will apply to you. That's not true of this book. There is a large *and diverse* community of people with concerns about weight and food. You have very different situations and problems. You have different stories. You have different genders, and in this arena, that is significant. So, while you're reading this book, you'll hear voices that *don't* sound like yours as well as voices that do. Listen to these other members of the community. They have something to tell you.

You'll also encounter suggestions that just don't click. It's important that you don't expect to relate to every word we say. After all, you're the one who needs to be in control here, not the diet center, not the diet gurus, and not us.

If you're a man, you're going to notice that some of this book seems to apply more to women than to you. Well, it does. Women in this society are under considerably more pressure than men to tailor their physical images to an ideal standard. And there are times when we must deal with the specific problems that arise from that pressure. Most of the book, however, can be useful to you as a person *and* as a person concerned about weight, even if you have to translate a few feminine pronouns.

We will, of course, provide the scientific and medical basis for our suggestions throughout the book. We won't rely on the anecdotal approach of the diet centers. But we have talked to a lot of people in preparing this book, and we will let you hear their voices. They are people who have taken control of their lives in this area. People like these:

> *Knowledge is power. Everybody always says that. But it's really true. I found out that the more information I had, the better I was able to take care of myself. And I don't just mean recipes and what has fat and that stuff. I mean understanding my body and what happens to women about that.*

> *It's exciting to eat now because there are so many new choices because of what I know now.*

> *I see these women at the health club and they're talking about how they haven't eaten in two days and I want to say, "Eat, please! Eat a lot."*

> *It was very painful for my husband to see me so angry with myself all the time. Since we've been together he's seen me through a range of forty pounds without batting an eye. But now he just loves seeing me be happy with myself.*

> *I'm not so mad at myself and the world. And I love exercise now as a celebration of my body instead of punishment.*

> *I still hate exercise, except walking. So I do my fifteen minutes of stair-stepping on a hassock while I'm watching "Barney Miller" reruns and I walk a couple of extra blocks to the bus stop.*

> *And if anybody tells me I should join an aerobics class, I just laugh at them, like I've always wanted to.*

> *I've lost thirty pounds and the most wonderful thing is I'm not on a diet. There's nothing to fall off of.*

> *I'm free. For the first time in my life I'm really free.*

PART I
Why America's Diet Industry Doesn't Work

Yes! Life is a banquet, and most poor sons of bitches are starving to death.

AUNTIE MAME
a.k.a. Patrick Dennis

1
Following the Script

It was beautiful and simple as all truly great swindles are.

O. HENRY

PHONE VOICE: Thank you for calling Weight Losers. May I help you?

HELEN: This is Helen Barnes. I saw your $19.95 special advertised. I'd like to know about it.

PHONE VOICE: Hi, (repeat caller's name), my name is Amanda. I'd be happy to give some general information about our program. (Use name), I'm so happy you called today. We offer a terrific program of prepared food, counseling, and support groups.

> *"They said the food was wonderful and easy. That I would be able to eat things I couldn't have on other diets. Well, if you think the freeze-dried hamburger resembles any piece of meat you have ever seen, think again."* Client: Nutri/System

> *"What you get is five or ten minutes of questions about how much water you drank, did you have your two servings of milk, etc., etc. Nothing that even resembled counseling."* Client: Nutri/System, Optifast

3

PHONE VOICE: We also have a maintenance program to teach you how to keep the weight off. And isn't that the most important thing? (pause)

"The diet is unrealistic, too rigid and difficult for anyone to follow unless they are really motivated and know that they are going to be weighed. No one could live this way." Counselor: Nutri/System

"I've tried them all. Some were easier than others. As long as I follow the rules, I lose. The second I leave, it starts coming back. I don't think I really expect to keep the weight off." Client: Weight Watchers, Jenny Craig, Nutri/System, TOPS

"One of my close friends was on the program. She was losing weight quickly. So I signed up. Now she's also fatter than when she started." Client: Optifast

"The lifetime dieter is our bread and butter money." Counselor: Nutri/System

PHONE VOICE: When you come in for your complimentary consultation we will answer all of your questions.

HELEN: Well, there are a couple things I need to know before I come in.

PHONE VOICE: (use name), how many pounds (do not say weight) would you like to lose? (acknowledge)

HELEN: I think I need to lose maybe twenty.

"Who decides the client's goal weight? We do, of course." Counselor: Diet Center

PHONE VOICE: (use name), I'd like to invite you to come in for a free consultation. At that time we'll explain the program to you in detail. We can see you now or later today, which would you prefer? (offer two times)

HELEN: I really can't afford more than $300 to do this. Do you think it will run more than that?

PHONE VOICE: (use name), we have several different kinds

of programs, starting as low as the special you called about. During your free consultation we will go through those programs with you and help you choose the one that meets your needs. (return to script)

"Lose your first ten pounds free. Sounds good. I had about seventeen pounds to lose according to the computer. Even though the first ten pounds came off in less than four weeks, that was still $360 worth of food. Hardly free. I had to purchase a program for the other seven pounds. They never came off, but it still cost me another $360 to struggle for four more weeks, plus a $99 Guaranteed Program fee. Eight hundred dollars is a lot of money for a free program." Client: Nutri/System

HELEN: Well, I know the food cost is separate, over the $19.95. Could you just tell me what I get each week and the price for the food?

PHONE VOICE: The cost of the food depends on your selection.

HELEN: Yes, I know, but—

PHONE VOICE: We have several menus and we will be glad to show them to you when you come in.

"I've only been on the program four weeks and I am already bored with the food. I would just like a piece of baked chicken. Would it be so terrible for me to have a piece of chicken?" Client: Nutri/System

"My dog would not eat that food." Client: Jenny Craig, Nutri/System

PHONE VOICE: (return to script) I can see you now or later today. Which is better for you?

HELEN: I have a family to feed as well, so the food price is very important to me. I need at least a ball park figure.

PHONE VOICE: I'd love to give you a better idea of the

cost. However, we want you to see the value of our program before you make your decision. I can see you now or later today. What time is better for you?

HELEN: I can come in about seven tonight.

PHONE VOICE: Great and the spelling of your last name . . . ?

HELEN: B-A-R-N-E-S.

PHONE VOICE: And a number you can be reached at by day . . . ?

HELEN: Five-five-five-two-five-three-four.

PHONE VOICE: And an evening number . . . ?

HELEN: It's the same.

PHONE VOICE: (use name), we are located at 2500 West Cermak. Are you familiar with the area? Okay, (use name), your appointment is for seven this evening. I'm really looking forward to meeting you. See you then.

"I was told when I bought this program it would help change my attitude about food permanently. It has. I feel guilty when I eat anything that was not okay on the program." Client: Weight Watchers, Nutri/System

"Yes, I was very successful on the Medifast. I got under 200 pounds for the first time in my life. When I left the program, I was 205 by the time I got to the corner of the street." Client: Medifast

"I'm not as upset about losing my gallbladder, as the fact that no one mentioned the medical risks." Client: Nutri/System

"I must be one of the lucky ones, the experience was pretty benign. I knew early on this program was not for me." Client: Optifast

2
Lose All the Weight You Want for $19.95

அ—⌐

Whatever they say they're going to do for you, don't believe them. They're just going to sell you the food. I know. I've tried all of them. They just sell you the food.

A DIET PROGRAM CLIENT

IN THE LAST decade, we have been getting closer and closer to a complete understanding of weight control. Research has never been more fruitful. Insights into physical, social, and emotional causes abound. Our grocery shelves are filling up with foods that can help us. Our bookstores have racks of books with sound advice.

And in the midst of all this, the diet industry thrives, ignoring every principle of healthy and successful weight control and charging customers hundreds of dollars for making them fatter.

In 1990, dieting was a $33 billion industry. That means sales larger than Eastman Kodak and Xerox combined. Or Wal-Mart together with Woolworth's. Or the gross national product of Ireland. Americans are spending more these days on diet pills, diet powders, diet books, and other diet dreams than on furniture for their houses, from sofas to sinks. We are desperate people looking for desperate remedies. And the diet centers stand ready, with open arms and reassuring faces, to assuage our fears. But what do they really offer?

Your first clue is their advertising. As you might suspect, advertisements for diet centers contain about as much information as ads for perfume. Their appeal is purely emotional. They all follow almost exactly the same format. They show you a person who has lost weight on their program, usually with photographs or home movies of what she looked like "before." Then they say that you can do the same. Sometimes there are five or six previously fat people with jazzy music and quick cuts from one to another. Sometimes there are family members saying how proud they are of Mom. Occasionally, a celebrity interviews the previously fat person. Jenny Craig sometimes varies this by appearing on screen herself, talking right to you, telling you about people she has helped, how moving it was to her and how much she wants to help you. (She has a high sincerity quotient and she uses it to the max.)

> We grew up founding our dreams on the infinite promise of American advertising. I still believe that one can learn to play the piano by mail and that mud will give you a perfect complexion.
>
> ZELDA FITZGERALD

These ads play on a lot of different emotions. They appeal to our dreams of being attractive and desirable. They pluck at our fears of being scorned or rejected. They make us believe that our husbands are ashamed of us and our children embarrassed by us. They are much more insidious than the pure sex appeal ads for mascara and nail polish. Somewhere deep inside, most of us know that thick lashes will not make us femmes fatales, but we genuinely fear that fifteen pounds of fat makes us repugnant.

In addition to all these things, the ads are selling instant gratification, the easy way to accomplish a difficult task. They are selling no work—no muss—no fuss. Just walk through our doors, they promise, and we'll turn your world right side up and put a smile on your face. You don't have to do anything except follow the rules. If you do follow the rules, you will be rewarded with a perfect body and all the perks that come with it. Love. Respect. Sex. Success. Self-esteem.

All this is a lot for a low $19.95 introductory offer.

Perfume ads sell sex. Diet center ads sell hope. The difference is, when you buy Obsession, you may not get sex, but at least you get something that smells good.

What you won't find in any advertisement for a diet program is information. The commercials will not tell you anything at all about:

- the details of the program itself
- what the program is going to cost you
- just how difficult the program really is
- what percentage of the diet center's customers these people in the commercials represent. Ten percent? Five percent? One percent?

The diet programs ask you to put your health in their hands. They also sell an expensive product, one that will cost you hundreds, even thousands, of dollars before you're through. And they tell you nothing. What's more, if, after watching the diet program commercial, you call the diet program to get information, you can't get it.

Go ahead. Try it. This is your first consciousness-raising exercise of this book. Look in the yellow pages for a big money diet center in your area —Jenny Craig, Nutri/System, Physicians Weight Loss, any of them. Call up, using a false name if it makes you feel safer, and try to get them to tell you what their program is going to cost. Roughly. Ball park figure. Ask them to tell you what the exercise component of the program consists of. Take a shot at getting a description of the available foods. Better yet, ask them how many people lose weight on their program.

They won't tell you. They'll get fired if they tell you.

There's a very good reason for this. They want to get you into the office for one of the most manipulative, exploitative, and effective sales gimmicks ever conceived. The Free Consultation.

They won't tell, but we will.

There are basically four types of programs. The first and most extreme, or rigid, of the programs is the very low-calorie liquid fast, such as Optifast and Health Management Resources. Next in order of restrictiveness is the food-inclusive diet center program, such as Jenny Craig. Third is the highly structured but not food-inclusive program. We will refer to it as the menu program. This group would include Diet Workshop, Diet Center, and Physicians Weight Loss Centers. And finally, we have those programs that are basically self-help support groups such as Overeaters Anonymous or TOPS (Take Off Pounds Safely).[1]

---

1. All of these programs change very frequently in order to remain competitive and afloat. Our information, which is from 1992 and early 1993, may not reflect the situation when you are reading the book or when you were in the program in, say, 1986. For instance, while this book was being written Nutri/System had three major diet format changes and several price increases. Both Nutri/System and Jenny Craig have dropped and readopted the phone script more than once. Diet Center previously required daily weigh-ins, but has compromised this policy because it was unrealistic for most of their clients.

This kind of shifting and changing is not unusual. It happens all the time in the food-inclusive programs and in the menu programs.

In addition, if the customers begin to disappear in the wake of increasing criticism, the programs will certainly make at least cosmetic changes to reclaim the market. Indeed, they already have made some changes. Promises of "quick" weight loss, for example, have disappeared from advertisements for virtually all the programs.

Also, there is wide variety from location to location. The degree to which policies, good or bad, are carried out depends on the character of the branch manager and the staff. The Diet Workshop leader in Des Moines may not run her program the same way as the group leader in Boston does.

The order in which the programs are presented is not arbitrary. The list begins with the type of program that has the most potential for creating problems.

THE LIQUID FAST

Optifast, Medifast, Health Management Resources

The basis of most of these programs is twelve to sixteen weeks of fasting on 400 or 500 calories a day's worth of powdered drink mix. All of these programs also claim to include a progressive "refeeding," "stabilization," and "maintenance" program, backed by support and counseling and medical supervision. These would be particularly important for the population that chooses fasting programs, a population that probably has the most difficulty with food and weight stability. If any group is likely to use food in a variety of emotional spheres, it is the group of overweight people who, after a number of battles and continual weight gain, turn to a fasting program as a last resort.

An example of this type of program is Health Management Resources, which offers the following: an initial medical evaluation, followed by weekly health monitoring; a weigh-in and blood chemistry biweekly; twelve weeks' worth of fasting, with nutrition provided by a 500-calorie-per-day supplement consisting of several packets of powder that are mixed with water. The protein in this plan is about forty-nine grams per day and is basically dried nonfat milk and egg whites. (There are also 800-calorie plans for those with less weight to lose.)

Patients are required to attend a weekly behavioral class in which nutritional education is also presented. The meetings cover exercise strategies and walking is recommended. This is one of the programs that claim to teach the patient how to return to the world of food through the

---

We include this note because what you read may not be your experience. It *is* the experience of the people we interviewed.

"refeeding phase." This is done by gradually weaning the patient from the packets as one meal at a time is replaced. The cost of the program is about $420 per month.

However, many of the Health Management Resources locations do not offer the full range of benefits, meaning that patients must either find and pay for their own counseling and nutritional education (in addition to the already alarmingly high cost) or do without.

Optifast is very similar. Its basic fasting supplement is 420 calories per day. There are weekly weigh-ins and medical checkups, but no individual counseling. As with Health Management Resources and virtually all of the other liquid fasting programs, emotional support, behavioral modification, nutritional education, lifestyle, and exercise are all "covered" by one weekly group meeting with twelve to fifteen other patients. The cost of the program is about $500 per month for about six months.

Most of these fasting programs have guidelines for acceptance into the program. At Optifast the policy is that a client be at least fifty pounds over his or her ideal weight or twenty pounds over and at medical risk. (It is not stated how ideal weight is determined.) Most of the other programs are less strict in their requirements.

Initially, some of the fasting programs were hospital-based. For that reason, health insurance often covers the cost. Today many of the programs are offered in clinics and through individual doctors, doctors who have no special training in bariatrics or the psychological issues of weight management and eating disorders and no more expertise in the problems of obesity than you would expect from any general medical practitioner.

Studies by groups such as Consumers Union, as well as our own interviews, indicate that fasting programs are difficult for most, and impossible for more than half, who start. Those who do follow through a twelve-week fast may lose large amounts of weight (twenty-five to fifty pounds), but most begin to regain as soon as food is reintroduced.

In her book *Diets That Work,* Deralee Scanlon, R.D., reviews the fasting approach.

. . . comparing dieters who consumed comparable low calorie amounts, the researchers found that those who ate rather than drank their calories felt more satisfied and complained less about hunger. This suggests that many people have a need to chew. Additionally, all rapid weight-loss diets burn not only fat, but some lean muscle tissue, potentially even the heart muscle; this is very unhealthy and can lead to sudden death. . . . All diets assume some risk, VLCDs [very low calorie diets] assume the most.

Italics are ours. Only a dietician would conclude that people are more satisfied with food than with reconstituted dry milk and egg white because they have a need to chew! Didn't this woman ever eat pizza?

FOOD-INCLUSIVE PROGRAMS

Jenny Craig, Nutri/System, Weight Watchers

Some programs claim to be "full service," providing food, counseling, nutritional education, and behavior modification. They exert a high degree of control over their clients.

Before going further, we need to clarify why Weight Watchers has been included in this group. A decade ago it would not have been listed here. In fact Weight Watchers has managed to remain sacrosanct, while all about it the other programs have been under attack. However, lately its halo has slipped.

Weight Watchers, like the other two programs, is focused on diet (food intake) and measured weight lost. It is a program of numbers. And from what we learned from former clients, far too many numbers. Today there are two programs. The first, "Mix and Match," is created primarily from the grocery shelves. However, Weight Watchers products are strongly encouraged for accuracy and convenience, especially since Heinz purchased the company. Weight Watchers is now a huge business and it does not make the money to pay for all those television commercials from its twelve-dollar-a-week fees. It makes it selling food. The support groups have become a marketing device, whatever their other purposes may be. And so, for our purposes, Weight Watchers is a food-inclusive program.

Even in "Mix and Match," clients focus a great deal of time and energy on keeping within very well-defined limits. This means measuring, knowing about dietary exchanges, counting calories, and eating at specified times. It is more restrictive than the average menu program. But there is also a second type of Weight Watcher program, called Personal Cuisine, which is a replica of Nutri/System and Jenny Craig in terms of weekly package food plans.

The major difference between Weight Watchers and the other food-inclusive programs at this point is that Weight Watchers does not even suggest that it offers counseling and the other presumably professional services offered by Nutri/System and Jenny Craig. (Also, its food does taste better.)

Since food is the major focus of this category of programs, let's start with that. Using Nutri/System's Crave Control Program as an example of a typical menu on a food-inclusive program, the following represents a typical day on the program. This is what you get for $77 per week:

BREAKFAST: 1 packet of instant oatmeal

LUNCH: 1 cup (envelope) chicken noodle soup
6 crackers

DINNER: Barbecue Beef and Potato Wedges

DESSERT: 1 chocolate chip cookie
(about 3 inches in diameter)

SNACK: 1 cup light microwave popcorn

Multiple vitamin

That $77 is not, however, your total food cost for the week. You have to supplement this food with stuff you buy yourself at the grocery store. At Nutri/System clients are instructed that they must supplement program food with the following:

BREAKFAST: 1 fruit (½ banana, apple, pear, or 12 grapes)
1 cup skim milk

LUNCH: salad vegetables, including celery, peppers, lettuce
diet beverage

DINNER: ½ cup cooked vegetable
1 fruit
1 cup skim milk

SNACK: 1 fruit

The cost of these additional ingredients is not large, but it's not negligible either.

The other two big diet center programs offer food packages similar to the Nutri/System menu described above. The difference is that Jenny Craig food is frozen, and the Weight Watchers Personal Cuisine is a combination of frozen, canned, and freeze-dried, while Nutri/System is mostly freeze-dried and must be reconstituted. Both programs also require the clients to supplement their food packages with food purchased at the grocery store.

To offer a basis of comparison, let's look at what similar food would cost if you bought it, ready-made and packaged, at the grocery store.

BREAKFAST: 1 packet of instant oatmeal

LUNCH: 1 envelope of chicken noodle soup
6 crackers

DINNER: Healthy Choice meat and potato dinner

DESSERT: 3 Entenmann's chocolate chip cookies (about 1.5 inches in diameter)

SNACK: 1 cup light microwave popcorn

Multiple vitamin

The total for this day, based on Chicago food prices, is about $4.25. Multiplied times seven, that would be $29.75 for a week. You would still be purchasing the extras you buy for any of these programs—fruit, vegetables, dairy (nonfat milk and/or yogurt), in some cases bread, and all of the condiments and beverages. Your actual cost would probably be lower than $29.75 because you would be incorporating these purchases in your family food purchases. In other words, your family can eat the fat-free cookies as well.

At most food-inclusive programs, food "extras" bring in a lot of revenue. The staff at Nutri/System has a prepared sales pitch for everything from salad dressings to flavored iced tea mix at $5.00 for four 1-quart packets. This is sold to clients as a water option (all programs require clients to drink eight glasses of water a day), though most nutritionists will tell you that iced tea is not a substitute for water. There are also a variety of snacks, flavored coffees, and even nonalcoholic "Wine Sparklers" made from fruit juice and soda water. Clients are given the idea that these products are vastly superior to the grocery equivalents, to the point of implying some magic in the ingredients. One staff member showed remarkable naïveté—or company loyalty—when she said to us, "I think the food has appetite suppressants, otherwise how could it work?"

As for what you are offered besides the food, the Weight Watcher routine is pretty well known. As we said earlier there is no pretense of professional support and informational services. All information, support, and behavioral change has to be a byproduct of the weekly meetings. These meetings can be led by anyone who has lost ten pounds on the program and been instructed by the company. A leader who regains her weight is relieved of her responsibilities.

Traditionally, the meetings have included public weigh-ins with vocal reactions from other group members about an individual's progress or lack thereof. We are told that, now, some Weight Watcher meetings have dispensed with these ritualized public weigh-ins and that comments on a member's failure to lose weight are discouraged. But weighing-in is still an important part of the meeting and the focus of the meeting is the talking about, supporting, rewarding, and deprecating members for the numbers that appear on the scale.

At Nutri/System and Jenny Craig, the initial orientation visit includes weighing-in, taking measurements, taking blood pressure, and going through some basic forms. The counselor gives you your first pep talk, explains the mechanics of how you are to eat on this program, and shows you how to order your food. At Jenny Craig, it is often the counselor who selects the menu.

After the first visit, your weekly appointment includes a weigh-in, ordering the next week's food, and a visit with the counselor for *about ten minutes*. During this visit she is expected to ascertain and record how well you are adhering to the program rules and your weight loss or gain, with comments. This is also the time when your counselor inquires about any problems you are having with the program and fixes those problems.

Clients are encouraged to go to weekly behavioral and motivational classes, but many centers have given up insisting that they be attended. Very often complaints about the leader make the manager back off rather than argue with a client. In the next chapter it will be clear why the classes are mostly ignored and as well as completely ineffective.

Nothing is done at any program with regard to exercise except advice that you should do it and at Nutri/System a video, at Jenny Craig an audio tape. Both these tapes are an additional expense. At Nutri/System, the video is included in the deluxe package. At Jenny Craig, it is part of an $80 to $90 package that also includes your behavioral conditioning lectures.

These programs will take anyone who feels a need to lose ten pounds, with some exceptions. Jenny Craig will not accept people with multiple food allergies or gluten intolerance. The three medical conditions that require a doctor's approval are diabetes, kidney disease, or heart disease. Nutri/System has somewhat higher standards. It will not accept pregnant women. A doctor's approval and a psychological counselor's approval are required for those who admit to a history of eating disorders. In addition to those with the three medical conditions listed for Jenny Craig, others who require a doctor's approval are people on antidepressants or diuretics.

At Weight Watchers, there is little or no monitoring of medical conditions. Those who admit to a complicating medical condition are advised to get their doctor's approval.

Nutri/System will accept clients eighteen years of age or, with a doctor's approval, at fourteen. At Jenny Craig, a doctor's approval is required for those eight to seventeen. Weight Watchers will accept ten-year-old children without a doctor's approval.

We will explain in the next chapter how these acceptance requirements are ignored or manipulated by various programs.

The major cost of these programs is the one we've already described—the food. The $70 to $80 a week you pay for food, multiplied by the number of weeks you remain in the program, is your basic figure.

Now, at your first meeting, Nutri/System and Jenny Craig are going to estimate that you will lose about two pounds a week. So, if you went in wanting to lose twenty pounds, your basic cost would be, say, $75 times ten, or $750.

However, there's a good chance your "goal weight" will be lower than what you had in mind when you went in for your Free Consultation. The computer programs are set to come up with unrealistically low goal weights for new clients. If you think you need to lose twenty pounds, the chances are the computer will say you need to lose thirty.

It's going to take you much longer to lose the last ten pounds than the first fifteen. You'll be fighting your body all the way, as we'll explain later. You don't want to abandon the goal weight stated on the contract or you'll forfeit your "weight maintenance refund." (That is the money refunded in some programs for losing weight and keeping it off for a year.) Also, your counselor will put pressure on you to remain in. So, you're likely to spend at least another month on the program trying to reach that goal, taking your cost up to over $1,000.

Your fee, in addition to the food cost, is highly variable. If you enter Jenny Craig or Nutri/System on a sale, you may pay $19.95 for your first four weeks. Then, if you want to stay, you will have to pay $200 to $300 for a "guarantee" program. The diet center will then guarantee to stick with you until you reach your goal weight, under certain conditions concerning attendance at meetings and appointments.

For your twenty pounds, you are now up to about $1,300.

Both these programs also offer lifetime memberships (a chilling thought for a diet program) for $300 to $400. At Nutri/System, a lifetime membership means that, at any time in your life, you can pay $49 and reenter the program, paying "only" for your food. Jenny Craig's program does not include a reentry fee.

At Weight Watchers, if you participate in the Personal Cuisine plan, you will pay about $70 per week for the food for the first three weeks, then $50 per week as you add two grocery store meals. So, assuming that you take ten weeks to lose twenty pounds, you have paid $560 for food. You will add to that your registration fee of $39 (including your first meeting) and about $12 per week for nine weeks. You are now up to $707.

Common complaints for most food-inclusive programs concern the quality of the food, its inconvenience, and its cost. People were also often shocked by the low quality of support systems such as counseling and classes.

"I couldn't believe it when the counselor told me not to exercise until several weeks into the program," says Fiona, a former Nutri/System client. "That is the one good habit I do almost every day."

Weight Watchers members are generally better satisfied, in part because they had no expectations of counseling or other education and because they believe that the program is "sound." However, they show no better results in losing weight or keeping it off.

THE MENU PROGRAMS

Diet Center, Physicians Weight Loss Centers, Etc., Etc., Etc.

There are a lot of menu programs around. They're much easier to set up than a food-inclusive program—you don't need food—so the small entrepreneur is likely to start here, with a storefront, a nutrition guide, and a copying machine.

This type of program provides structure and accountability, but there is no food sold except company specialty items such as salad dressings and food supplements. Clients are provided with menus, which they use when purchasing grocery store food. The main selling point for these programs is intensive one-on-one counseling and nutritional education. They make a virtue of not providing a food package by saying that you will learn better how to shop for and feed yourself.

The menu program is probably the most difficult to describe as a group. Each has its own eccentricities. For instance, some restrict whole groups of food. Others require daily visits to the diet center and daily weigh-ins. The best we can do is give you some of the common features and then describe one of the more popular programs, Diet Center, in more detail.

Most of the diets are low calorie (1,000 to 1,200 is average) and low fat and *totally prohibit* sugar. They are very specific with regard to amounts and combinations of foods. Some offer a combination of food and formula. Support services include longer and more frequent counseling sessions than in the food-inclusive programs, though the counselors are unlikely to have any significant training in psychology or nutrition.

Diet Center currently offers a program called *Exclusively You,* which uses a computer to generate "personalized" diets and exercise programs. They are based on a variety of factors, such as age, gender, and family history.

This is very similar to having a computer personalize your makeup selection at a department store counter. The diet itself has four phases: conditioning (two days), reducing, *Sta-bil-lite*, and maintenance. Caloric intake ranges from 1,000 to 2,000 calories a day. A typical Diet Center day's menu might look like this in the reducing phase for a 160-pound woman.

6 to 7 ounces of protein

2 to 3 fruit servings (½ banana is a serving)

5 to 6 vegetable servings (3 must be raw)

2 to 4 servings of grains

1 or 2 servings dairy

2 teaspoons of oil

The actual menu would specify foods, not just types.

Program costs are based on the number of pounds you are going to lose, which is usually determined by a computer, as it is in all the programs. The Diet Center enrollment and registration fee will be from $52 to $79. The weekly fee will be from $37 to $53. Therefore, in our scenario of losing twenty pounds in ten weeks, the fees would be from about $422 to $609, plus a maintenance program that lasts one year for $110. The total, therefore, is from $532 to $719 *without food.*

SELF-HELP SUPPORT GROUPS

Tops, Overeaters Anonymous

Generally speaking these groups are based on the ideas of one individual who had success in modifying food behavior and/or weight by working with a small support group. The program may consist of very general guidelines like TOPS or, like some OA groups, have a very rigid structure. A great deal depends on the particular leader and the personalities of those in the group.

Some of the former OA members we talked to indicated that they had gone to groups that encouraged strict abstinence, meaning, not starvation, but three healthy meals each day with no snacks, no sweets, and no exceptions. We even talked to one woman who, after being on the program for five years and having to call from a restaurant for permission to substitute peas for broccoli, felt the need to be deprogrammed.

But other people described the program as much looser and very much focused on mutual support. Some of them had been meeting with the same support group for ten or fifteen years and considered their fellow members to be close personal friends.

Throughout the second half of this book we emphasize the enormous value of working in a support group. Going through many of the processes necessary to make a meaningful change is greatly aided by a good support system. This means a place where you have the safety to say what you feel, be who you are, and find encouragement from the group for your personal goals. These groups *may* serve that purpose. However, before committing to one, it would be a good idea to read the guidelines to choosing a group that we present in Chapter 13, "Getting Help."

The cost of these groups may be no more than a minimal weekly donation to cover the cost of the meeting place and coffee. Usually these groups meet in churches, YMCAs, or community centers.

3
Why Diet Programs Don't Work

*I've weighed more than 200 since I was
in high school. I've been on all of them—
Weight Watchers, Slim Fast, Jenny Craig,
TOPS. . . . But as soon as I gain back the
first few pounds, it's over.*

DIET PROGRAM VETERAN

WHEN WE INTERVIEWED diet program counselors for this
book, we asked them to tell us how many of their clients
they estimated to be repeaters, people who had previously
been on their program or another one. The estimates of
the counselors ranged from a low of 70 percent to 80 or
90 percent. One counselor said, "Almost all of them. I'd
say easily 90 percent." Another said, "We couldn't stay
in business if it weren't for the repeats!"

This does not describe a lasting solution to the problem
of weight control.

One counselor at Nutri/System said, "After I had been
at the program a couple of years, I was astonished at the
people I was seeing over and over again. Sometimes, when
they came back, I couldn't resist asking them why. What
went wrong? The answer was, 'I have to come here. Without the diet I have no willpower or self-control.' "

Even more disturbing were the responses from the clients themselves, women who knew they would be doing

this over and over. When one Nutri/System client was asked why she had repeated the program so often, she said it was the only way she could survive. Come in several times a year, lose twenty to thirty pounds and go home to gain it back. This at least kept her "sort of even." She, like most diet center clients, believes that the failure is hers. And the diet centers encourage this belief.

The idea of blaming the customer when the program fails is one hitherto limited to faith healing, but the diet centers get away with it. To begin with, whose fault is it if a customer fails to complete a weight loss program? The diet centers say the blame lies with the customer. She simply didn't have the persistence—the minimal persistence, they suggest—that anyone who really wants to lose weight should have. When they are selling the program, they say, in essence, "Come to us and you won't need willpower." When they are justifying their failures, they say, "What did you expect? You just didn't have enough willpower."

> There's a strong aroma of sawn lady about this.

> JOSEPHINE TEY

But suppose a customer—through sheer will or compulsive behavior—manages to get through and lose weight. Who is to blame when she does not keep it off? Again, the diet centers imply, it's her fault. She goes back to eating "bad food" and so, of course, she gains weight. There is no recognition of the fact that the deprivation diet has seriously altered the customer's metabolism and ability to use food. One counselor we interviewed described a woman whose body had been so altered by dieting that she now gained weight on 600 calories a day. That's one honey-glazed doughnut and a glass of milk. The customer is very likely to end up a year after the program not only having regained the weight she lost, but having added to her weight because of her metabolic shift. She starts the diet weighing 150. A year later, she weighs 160. The program has helped to nudge her body further in the direction of being a fat creator rather than a fat burner. It has made the situation worse, not better.

This is why the diet programs use anecdotal advertising—individual testimonials, usually from people who have just completed the program. Nutri/System defends its program with a study based on twenty clients who managed to keep off the weight for fifteen months. All twenty of those people were being used in Nutri/System television commercials at the time, a motivation that most clients obviously don't have. The problem would, of course, be serious enough if the diet centers were simply ineffective. But the situation is far worse than that. People who are desperate are being sabotaged by the companies they turn to for help.

Okay, the programs don't work for most people. But could they work for me? At all? Even a little bit?

That's the question that keeps people coming back, even when they don't buy the glitzy commercials, even when they manage to see through the sympathetic "counselors." There's always the hope that, if you work hard enough at it and are good enough, it just might work for you, even if it doesn't work for anyone else. So let's look at that question.

THE PHYSICAL REALITY

Put aside for the moment the fact that diet programs *don't* work and let's look at whether there is any chance that they *can*. To begin with, what do the diet programs offer? As we've seen, that varies from program to program, but not very much. They differ in services, but not in concept. First and foremost, the programs offer diets. Liquid diets, program diets, menu diets. And diets don't work.

You've probably heard that before. But did you believe it? If you're like most people with a history of dieting, you didn't. First, because you've actually lost weight on diets and second, because you *can't afford to believe it.*

Second things first. If weight is an issue for you, if you feel that your eating is out of control, the only time you feel good about yourself is when you're dieting. It is your only hope. You can't afford to believe the books called *Diet Is a Four Letter Word* or *Diets Don't Work*. They leave you feeling powerless in the face of your most dreaded enemy. So, no matter how logical their arguments are, you can't afford to believe them.

Well, we're making you a promise here. If you read the second half of this book, we will give you other methods, *besides dieting,* that can work for you. Right now, try to believe that statement and go on to the other reason you don't believe that diets don't work.

You've lost weight on diets. We've all done it. Diets can take weight off ... in the very short run. But the weight comes back. It's difficult to imagine a doctor saying to a patient, "Yes, I can remove that wart. Of course, it will almost certainly come back, and probably even larger. Is that a problem?" But that, in essence, is the only prognosis that program diets can honestly offer.

> But if one doesn't have a character like Abraham Lincoln or Joan of Arc, a diet simply disintegrates into eating exactly what you want to eat, but with a bad conscience.
>
> MARIA AUGUSTA VON TRAPP

Deprivation dieting guarantees the return of lost weight, for both emotional and physiological reasons. By a deprivation diet, we mean one that significantly and suddenly lowers caloric intake or, as Dr. Jean Mayer puts it in his *Diet and Nutrition Guide,* "any diet that is out of step with your lifestyle and preferences." And anyone with the nutritional and bariatrics training that diet centers claim for their employees *knows* this to be the case. Indeed, the training manual for one of the largest diet centers in the country states it very clearly. "Unfortunately, when you go on a diet, your body doesn't know you are trying to lose weight; it just knows it's not getting enough food so its natural reaction is for the metabolism to slow down and use less energy." This statement is used by the diet center to explain why a dieter might hit a "plateau." In fact, it explains why most people can't lose weight on the programs and those who manage to complete weight loss programs are doomed to eventual failure.

Depending on who you are and how much you move around, your body needs a certain amount of fuel just to keep going. If you take in significantly more fuel than your body can use it is stored as fat. If you take in a lot less fuel, your body burns off some of the previously stored fat. This is where the logic of low-calorie dieting evolved. If you cut back the fuel/food consumption enough, you'll burn the stored fat and lose weight. Except . . .

The exception occurs when you consistently let your fuel/calories dip below the point needed to sustain life— go on a low-calorie diet. Then, your body begins conserving energy, in order to try to preserve the weight your body thinks it ought to be. It slows your metabolism, becoming more fuel efficient. We'll go into this in much more detail in Part Two, but these are the basics.

You know the woman in your diet program, the one who is about forty and about forty pounds above "her goal"? She claims she sticks to the program religiously and still cannot lose weight. Right.

Well, she's probably telling the truth. She's been on every diet under the sun. Most recently she lost fifty pounds on a liquid fast containing about 800 calories a day. What her body learned on the liquid fast was how to survive on 800 calories. Now the new diet program she's on allows 1,200 calories, so her body is taking that "extra" 400 calories and trying to store it. The only way she can keep from *gaining* weight on her current diet is to avoid some of the recommended food and go to aerobic dance class several times a week. This is a classic example of what happens to human metabolism when it is under threat of starvation.

The other thing that happens when you don't eat enough is that you get hungry. Very, very hungry.

Yes, binge eating after a diet (or even during one) is perfectly normal behavior. It is not simply rebellion or a response to psychological deprivation, although that would be enough. It is hunger striking back. "Hunger does accumulate," say William Bennett, M.D., and Joel Gurin in *The Dieter's Dilemma,* "there is really no question of that. Dieters demonstrate it. . . . Any laboratory rat will demonstrate it: Take away its rations until the animal loses twenty or thirty grams, then give it free access to food and it will eat very earnestly until it has restored the missing fat."

Bennett and Gurin give many examples of how cumulative hunger works, including one about "the ricers." The ricers were a group of obese patients put on the famous Duke University brown rice diet. One ricer described her most triumphant moment: when she stole a nineteen-pound turkey from the hospital kitchen, smuggled it into her room, and by three in the morning had consumed the whole bird and disposed of the remains. Because the turkey was freshly cooked and she had to hide it under her nightgown, she suffered an unpleasant burn, but she had no regrets.

This woman was not crazy. She was under the influence of a physical impulse as strong as any a human being is likely to experience. It was her body's impulse to stay alive, to maintain her weight.

So, what is the answer to our original question, "Can diet programs work?" The answer is no. The only way a 1,200 calorie reducing diet can work is if it is also low fat, is accompanied by exercise—we'll go into that later—and *if you stay with it for the rest of your life.* The moment you go back up to 1,500 calories or change the amount of fat in your diet, the weight will come back.

What's more, if you can't stay on the diet for the rest of your life, you will almost certainly end up worse off than when you started. Physically, a series of diets makes you fatter. If, after the first few diets, you only go back to your original weight, don't be fooled. Today's number on the scale is not the whole picture. You *are* becoming fatter. Each time you put the weight back on, you are adding fat cells. And they never go away.

· So the fat get fatter, and the lean get anything they want on the menu. Jenny Craig can tell you all day that you should think of your diet center the way you think of your dentist or your hairdresser. You know, lose the weight, gain it back, come on in and lose it again. The fact is that, if you do, you'll end up a lot fatter a couple of years down the road. You don't want to add any little fat cells to your genetically programmed stores. And every time you gain weight back from a diet, you do.

Physically, deprivation dieting doesn't work. And the people who run the diet centers know this. *Jenny knows it.* This information is not new. It has been around for years.

THE DOUBLE WHAMMY

Psychologically, the picture is just as bad.

When we talk about deprivational diets, we are talking about anything that encourages you to ignore or deny hunger, toss your old habits in the garbage and eat a lot of stuff that isn't what you really want to eat. That doesn't work, either. Not only does this make sense, but it is being shown to be true by the research community.

Optifast and the other fasting programs are seriously deprivational both physically and psychologically, for anyone. "I went off the fast, ate my first meal, I couldn't stop," says Kay, who has been through Optifast twice. "I think that meal lasted about a week." This is not an unusual reaction to fasting.

For most people, the food-inclusive diets and menu diets are less serious physically but very serious psychologically. And the physical element *is* there. For larger people, even the food-inclusive diets have a very powerful physical effect.

One Nutri/System customer recently exclaimed to her counselors, "Can't you people see that no one who weighs more than 300 pounds can exist on this food? I've been having crazy, violent feelings all week. There were times

I felt like I could kill someone. Look at my hands. They're still shaking. Why don't you warn people about this?''

Kim, an employee of one of the diet programs, found her perspective changing when she became her own client.

"I've been thinking lately about smoking again," she told us. "It sounds terrible. It was a battle to quit after thirty-five years. In the year since I've quit, though, I've gained more than twenty pounds, I'm sure. I wonder if it's worth it. I've never been fat. And, boy do I feel fat right now. I was a size twelve from the time I was in high school. I'm lucky if I can wear a sixteen. I didn't have this much trouble with my weight over two pregnancies. It's driving me crazy to be struggling over what to eat, what not to eat. I'm thinking like all my diet-crazed friends."

When we interviewed Kim, we thought we were going to be talking about her experience as a diet program staff member. And then, over coffee, she spilled out all this frustration. She was never in touch with client thinking until she gave up smoking about a year ago. But when she started trying to get rid of her post-smoking weight, she learned fast.

For a few months she tried the diet center program. Even though she had seen all the repeats and failure, like everyone else she hoped things would be different for her. Besides it was convenient and they gave her a discount.

Because she was a "natural thin," and someone who had not dieted before, the weight came off rather easily. There were weeks when clients who had long diet histories couldn't lose an ounce, while Kim consistently dropped at least two pounds. The weight came off steadily, but she would be the first person to admit staying on the program was not easy. She was hungry most of the time. After the first couple of weeks she really began to crave her one favorite snack, potato chips.

Again because Kim had not had a previous problem, she occasionally still had the potato chips and lost weight. The other significant change Kim made was that she began to walk regularly. She decided she would walk to work and home at least four days a week. The walk was about twenty-five minutes, from home to office.

After a couple of months of this routine Kim had lost most of the weight. The problem was that now she felt deprived and unable to deal with food in what she calls "any rational, normal way." In just a few weeks of "trying to live normally again" the weight had started to return. She was miserable.

And now she was seriously considering going back to cigarettes.

In two separate studies recently, the results showed that the majority of successful weight losers had created their own plans.

That's what works.

And diet programs, whatever they tell you on television, don't help you do that. If they did, they'd go broke.

> *One of the most striking differences between a cat and a lie is that a cat has only nine lives.*

> MARK TWAIN

To sum up, diet programs don't work as a cure for obesity. They don't even have a lasting effect on minimal overweight. They are based on ideas that are long out of date. They don't work for a variety of physical and psychological reasons. And, everyone involved knows— or should know—they don't work.

The industry top management may or may not keep success/failure data. (You can be damned sure they keep track of how many "weight maintenance refunds" they hand out.) They certainly are not about to publish numbers on the failure rate. But the personnel interviewed knew that the customers are repeats, that only a small fraction of those who start these programs lose any weight at all and that virtually all those who do lose weight gain it back after they leave the program. Everyone is aware of the number of "closed files" in back offices.

Mute acknowledgment of this cyclical failure is the appearance of lifetime membership programs such as Nutri/System's Premier Program. The sales representative presents the program this way. "We all know there are those stressful periods in life when you are bound to gain some weight back—moving, new job, a pregnancy. With the Premiere Membership you can come back for our full services as often as you want, with no new initiation fee." What she's thinking is, "Chances are if she's been dieting all these years, she'll be in for the full program every year."

Chances are she's right.

4
The Food

I never had to pay attention. I think I almost resent even trying after years of watching my mother, then my wife, obsess about food. It may be part of the reason I'm a real junk food addict. I refuse to do anything but go into a diet center where they just hand me the food.

DIET PROGRAM CLIENT

WHAT'S THE FIRST thing you think after you think diet?

Well . . . food.

That's right, food. What am I going to eat? How much am I going to eat? Is it going to taste good? Am I going to be happy enough with it to keep going? Tell me about the food.

Food is the focus of any commercial diet program. Providing you with food—or a food plan—is how they say they will make this difficult task easier. They will take the thinking, and in some cases, the preparation out of your hands. They will do it all for you. But what is it they will do?

Most diet programs claim to offer a nutritionally sound diet. Most dieticians would disagree. Diet menus range from 800 to about 1,200 calories a day. According to the National Research Council's *Recommended Dietary Allow-*

ances, it is virtually impossible to get all the nutrition you need from less than 1,500 calories a day. For years, Nutri/System advertised that its program met the dietary guidelines of groups such as the American Heart Association and the American Medical Association, *in spite of repeated protests by those groups.* They didn't give it up until they were faced with a Connie Chung interview. Then they promised to be good.

But even if a diet is nutritionally sound, it can't work if *you* can't eat that way.

RIGIDITY AND RESTRICTIVENESS

Oddly enough, the issue of food takes on importance in the fasting programs *by its absence.* In this sort of program, clients do not choose or eat any food for a minimum of three months. Whatever happens to their weight during that time, there's going to be a problem when it ends. What do the program's designers actually expect from a 250-pound individual—one who was previously a regular customer of America's fast food emporiums—when food is once more an option? Is it likely that someone who thought a twelve-ounce steak and a large order of fries a great dinner will find three ounces of lightly seasoned broiled fish with green beans appealing? Or even consider this a choice?

> Food is an important part of a balanced diet.
>
> FRAN LEBOWITZ

To counter this obvious flaw, the fasting programs insist that they wean clients gradually from liquid meals and, at the same time, provide them with adequate educational backup about sensible eating. They claim that by the end of the refeeding phase of the program, clients are sophisticated in the fine points of healthful eating.

This claim for the efficacy of educating clients did not hold up in our interviews. Almost all of the clients who had been on fasting programs said that the return to food represented a great problem. Again, like the anorexic, they felt guilty eating anything, certainly anything that tasted good. Most said they started to gain the weight back almost as soon as the fasting ended. Some of them continued to go to weekly support meetings for a while. But after one or two breakdowns (a candy bar or fried chicken) all of their efforts ended. Within a year or less they went back to their prediet eating habits and were close to their prediet weight.

In the food-inclusive programs, the problem is less dramatic but just as pervasive. Lasting success on someone else's diet is almost nonexistent. Fact. The diet programs may tell you that you won't even notice you're dieting, but if you're not eating what you want, you'll notice. You may look at the program menu, or the exchanges, and think, "three sensible meals and *snacks.* That's not deprivational." But if it's not the way you have been eating, if it's not the way you like to eat, it's deprivational. If what you want the second you open your eyes is coffee and a doughnut, if that's what you dream about on the diet, and that's what you go right back to after the diet, two months on wheat toast and skim milk is going to be worse than useless.

This is not just some kind of health pep talk. It's been proven time and again, in study after study.

As soon as you are denied your choices and natural instincts, there is a tension—a tension that, if extreme and frequent, becomes an obsession. All diets that you did not personally design from your own preferences, that you did not test and ease into, are deprivational and *they won't last.* They may have been based on sound theories of human physiology and nutrition, but they have no relationship to your likes and life and, sooner or later, you will fall off of them.

*The trouble about always trying to pre-
serve the health of the body is that it is*

> *so difficult to do without destroying the*
> *health of the mind.*
>
> G. K. CHESTERTON

Just look at the logic of the diet center program. In order to lose weight, they say, you must be deprived suddenly and drastically and for an extended period of time. And then, gradually, you will be weaned back to normal eating. This is like a health club that, on your first day, puts you on a program of jogging six miles a day, working out on the Nautilus machines at elevated weight and repetition levels, and climbing the Stairmaster for an hour at a time, with the reassurance that, after a while, you will be gradually returned to normal levels of exercise.

It doesn't work that way. That's why about half of the clients of food-inclusive programs *don't come back for the second week*. They pay their fees, they buy their first week's groceries, and then, like a health club customer who can't keep up with the six miles a day and the Nautilus, they just don't come back.

"Okay, I tried for one week. This is ridiculous," said Rima to a counselor who was trying to keep her on the program. "I sell real estate. I am either in the car all day driving around, or taking a customer to lunch or eating at very odd times. You told me this would work into my lifestyle. This was supposed to make things easier. But I don't think I can do another week."

That's half of them. The rest stick it out longer, until about the fifth week. Up to that point, dieters will say that everything is fine, no problem. Then, suddenly, they fall off with a bang ... or a binge. Many more clients leave at about that point. Those who stay experience greater and greater difficulty at keeping with the program. The majority gradually fall away, before reaching their goal weight.

Clients who don't like breakfast run into resistance when they ask about reordering their food day. (Yes, we know you have read over and over that your diet problems begin with skipping breakfast. We don't think so, and neither do other experts who work with compulsive dieters/

compulsive eaters.) Indifference to personal choice is also evident in programs that follow a no-substitution policy. The Nutri/System plan, for example, once included a snack plus *two sweet desserts*. Clients complained that they had gotten out of the habit of eating sweets and would prefer fruit for dessert. Their complaints were ignored for a long time, while the company defended their "necessity of sweet foods." Later, in an economy measure, the sweets were replaced by fruit bought by the client. (The price of the program was not lowered to reflect this change.)

The counselors we interviewed had their own comments.

"Are you kidding?" said one. "Some of [the clients] never come back after the first week. And believe me, the center tries. We call clients daily when they miss an appointment. It's revenue. About seventy-five dollars is lost if they don't come for their appointment."

"The majority of people last four to six weeks," said another, "probably because almost all of them drop eight to ten pounds initially, just from the change in diet and water loss. Once it slows down for a couple of weeks, they get discouraged and go. Often we see them back in about three months, heavier than when they were here before."

"I never thought about it before," another told us, "but I'd say maybe 10 percent get through the program, sometimes not to their goal weight. They just can't stay with the diet any longer. Some start gaining again so we let them go into maintenance."

QUALITY AND QUANTITY

Another counselor said to us, "Get real. How long do you think people can live on this freeze-dried food?" And a woman who worked for the same program laughed as she hid her Dunkin' Donuts bag and said, "I couldn't live on that stuff if you paid me."

These are not unusual complaints. Many people find the food unpalatable or the selections undesirable. Even more clients find the portions unacceptable. One woman told her counselor that, in order to have enough for dinner, she poured her entree, about two thirds of a cup of beef stew, over a sixteen-ounce bag of frozen vegetables. (She felt guilty, because the program limited vegetables to one-half or one-cup servings.) Another begged to be allowed to replace her required eight-ounce glass of skim milk with nonfat cottage cheese because she had always hated milk. Permission was refused. One woman asked the counselor if she had ever *seen* the disgusting ham packed in gelatin that she was being expected to eat.

> The effect of eating too much lettuce is "soporific."
>
> BEATRIX POTTER

"I have to tell you the truth," said Stan to his Nutri/System counselor, "by afternoon I've eaten most of my food for the day. I start working construction at 5 A.M. That turkey sandwich and a piece of fruit just doesn't do it. I wind up eating the dinner and snacks in the afternoon. What am I supposed to eat from three until I go to sleep at eleven? Instead of diet food, I give in to running out for a hamburger."

Apologizing to her counselor, Nell explained, "I feel really guilty that I couldn't stay with the program 100 percent. There were some foods I mentioned that I don't like. They put them in my food bag anyway. So I just throw them away and eat something else. Even popcorn for dinner is better than cardboard hamburger."

It's just too hard to eat what you don't want and don't like and don't even have enough of.

LEARNING TO EAT

A recent *Glamour* magazine article stated, "The chief advantage of premeasured foods is that they teach portion control and remove the burden of making choices." The first of those claims is wrong and the second is *not* an advantage. People do not learn to control their own portions by having someone else do it. And the "burden" of making choices is what every person concerned about weight has to learn to shoulder.

Diet programs, from liquid fasts all the way through nonprofit support groups, claim to educate people. But you can ask any teacher or any mother whether a child learns *anything* by having someone else do it for her.

After all, there is no "right" way to eat. If you look at the many diet programs, they differ greatly in what the client is expected to eat and not to eat. In the programs that require clients to purchase food, there is a significant difference in the percentage of fat allowed in the diet (from 15 to 24 percent). There are also major differences in the kind of carbohydrates clients can eat. Some programs are so restrictive that they do not permit even starchy vegetables in any quantity. Other programs take a different tack, providing sugary desserts so the client will not feel deprived. If any one of these was really "right," somebody would be losing weight out there and keeping it off. And they're not.

> I generally avoid temptation unless I
> can't resist it.
>
> MAE WEST

Those programs that do not sell food pride themselves on allowing free selection of grocery store food. At the same time they hand clients a very precise menu. For instance, when a counselor at Diet Center was asked what the program restrictions were, she pointed out "the best thing about Diet Center is that you get to buy your own foods at the grocery." "What are the guidelines?" we inquired. "Oh, they are very loose. We simply ask clients to keep to low fat, no sugar, and low sodium." "That means clients can have a free selection of complex carbohydrates, like bread, pasta, etc.," we responded. Absolutely not said the counselor. "They are allowed one slice of Wasa Crisp-bread a day." If this is free choice, the person who's free sure isn't you.

It is probably a fair assumption to say that the creators of the top diets—Weight Watchers, Jenny Craig, Diet Workshop—had roaring successes on their own diets. But the diets are theirs, not yours. What they find pleasurable, or at least acceptable, for a lifetime may seem like the Spanish Inquisition to you. What Richard Simmons does has obviously worked out splendidly for him, but you are not Richard Simmons.

In a nutshell, commercial diet programs are doomed to failure because, no matter how well designed theoretically, they are not made to *your* design. They require you to eat without regard to your body's needs and preferences and to obey a set of externally imposed guidelines. And that just won't work in the long run.

5
Support Services

*Where are all those great counselors they
talk about on TV? Mine just wanted to
know if I drank my water.*

DIET PROGRAM CLIENT

*SO DIETS DON'T work, and the food's not great. Is that all
these programs have to offer?*

Well, they claim it isn't. But the claims don't hold up
very well.

In recent years, diet centers have attempted to appear
more responsible by saying they offer the elements health
professionals have suggested should be in a weight loss
program—healthful eating, exercise, counseling, education,
and behavioral conditioning. But their paper virtue simply
doesn't translate into practical strength. Deprivation diets
still remain by far the biggest emphasis. In large part this
is because selling their own brands of low-calorie food is
the greatest source of income for the three giants in the
field—Weight Watchers, Nutri/System, and Jenny Craig.

The manager of one outlet told us that, in his office,
the initial fees would not be enough to pay salaries and
overhead—if all the customers remained in the program,
that is. Most of the money, he pointed out, was made on
the food, which has an enormous markup. In this company,
as in most food-inclusive programs, any counselor who

gives a customer permission to vary in the slightest degree from the prescribed diet—made up of the diet center's food—is called on the carpet for costing the company profits.

Weight Watchers has a better reputation in this area. However, as *Fortune* points out, ''While dieticians praise Weight Watchers for not pushing its own brands too forcefully in its classes, the message gets across anyway. Handouts at lectures often include coupons, and staying on the complex diet can require such tedious calculations that many dieters just stock up on Weight Watchers food instead. As a result, Heinz [which owns Weight Watchers] sold $780 million of the Weight Watchers brand last year, 20 percent more than in 1987. Heinz Chairman Anthony O'Reilly expects the same dramatic growth over the next five years. By the mid-nineties, *Weight Watchers products will outsell all Heinz's other food products* [our italics].''

Even the menu programs usually sell powders, drinks, salad dressings, and other supplements. But food sales are not the only reason that diet is emphasized in the merchandising of weight loss. The fact is that diet programs are selling *magic,* in the same sense that Dr. Sleazebottom's Traveling Medicine Show did in the days before the FDA. Sometimes the magic is special food. Sometimes it may only be the particular combinations and permutations of carrots, broccoli, and grapefruit listed on the diet sheets. But dieting can be made to seem a miracle cure in a way that exercise, healthful eating, and emotional support cannot.

The diet is where the magic is. The diet is where the money is. As a result, the rest of the program is shortchanged. And any chance that the programs might educate you, raise your consciousness, permanently change your weight and improve your way of eating is lost.

COUNSELING

Psychological counseling is potentially a very useful service. But there isn't much of it going around the diet industry.

In the fasting programs, individual counseling should be an absolute priority, for a number of reasons.

First, for a person who is carrying a considerable amount of body fat, going without food is going to cause a very serious starvation response. Asking someone simply to "deal with" overwhelming feelings of hunger is, at best, unrealistic. It isn't going to happen, not until that person reaches a state that many people have described to us as "free of food." In other words, fasters will eventually develop a condition similar to anorexia, though only temporarily. Before that, they will be devoured by hunger. Afterward, they will be completely out of touch with their bodies' needs. *They shouldn't be doing this alone.*

> *Desire to have things done quickly pre-*
> *vents their being done thoroughly.*

> CONFUCIUS

Second, the program is asking people who almost certainly have developed strong emotional connections with food and eating to deny those connections. What happens to the emotions that are now not finding expression or release in food?

They burst out all over, that's what. Fasters report bouts of anger, depression, and extreme frustration. Eating is a survival skill. (We'll talk more about that in Part Two.) Rob a person of that skill and emotional survival becomes shaky. This is a problem for a professional psychologist or psychiatrist, one who specializes in eating problems or disorders. Most professionals agree this is a very specialized area of counseling.

So what counseling do the fasting programs provide? As we've seen, they offer group meetings that are often so ineffectual the patients fail to attend. That's it. One woman who enrolled in a "medically supervised" fasting program described her experience this way. "I was seen by a doctor for the initial evaluation only and blood workup. After that I was seen by a very pleasant lady who just weighed me, smiled if I lost weight, and praised me like a child. If I did not lose, she would reprimand me. The weekly group behavior meetings were a waste of time. They didn't tell me anything I didn't know before the fast. I would usually leave very depressed.''

As a psychologist with a specialty in this area, Diane has often had clients who were referred to her by a fasting program or by the insurance company that is paying for the program. In other words, while the patient is getting her powdered milk and egg and her weigh-in from the hospital for thousands of dollars, she has to go elsewhere for the one thing she needs most.

In the food-inclusive programs, the situation is even worse. Counseling usually consists of a ten-minute question-and-answer session that accompanies the weigh-in. And its primary purpose is *not* to provide emotional support to the client. The session is designed to protect the center against law suits and to provide material for market research.

When the customer comes in for counseling, the counselor asks her questions about her health and about how she is sticking to the diet. If, in the future, she suffers any medical problems as a result of the diet, the center can refer to the records to prove that the problems were not mentioned by the customer, *even though the counselor asked.* Also, if the client later claims to have developed a problem, the center can refer to any variations from the diet to absolve itself from responsibility.

Where food is sold or supplements handed out, records must be kept, and that's how the little time available is used. In our interviews with counselors in food-inclusive programs, this was a great area of frustration. In response to a question in our interviews, ''Are there any particular features of this program that you thought were helpful or especially bad?'' the lack of counseling time came up again and again. One counselor from a nationwide diet center said, ''I don't care if a client comes in sobbing her eyes out. There is no time to talk to her about what's wrong. Just ask her the questions on the tracking sheet and go on.''

The company also uses the information garnered in these sessions to determine what sells and what doesn't.

There is virtually no value in these sessions to the client's emotional well-being. Indeed, they are often filled with recriminations for insufficient weight loss and with reproaches for failure to stick closely enough to the diet. They can end up doing more harm than good.

Part of the problem is that most of the "counselors" are not qualified to counsel. The image presented, carefully and deliberately, by most diet programs is one of a scientifically based, medically sound approach to weight loss administered by "qualified" personnel. When you walk in the door at Nutri/System or Physicians Weight Loss Centers, for example, you'll see people walking around in white lab coats. Certainly the very name *Physicians* Weight Loss Center suggests medical supervision. At various diet program centers, you will be assigned to someone with a title like "Nutritional Counselor" and be given the impression that you are in the hands of a person with special training in nutrition or weight loss psychology.

Does this image have any basis in fact?

A House subcommittee headed by Congressman Ron Wyden was disturbed to find out that it does not. Not one of the centers investigated was under the supervision of full-time medical professionals who would be qualified to recognize and deal with possible health problems.

And those people in the white coats are not just failing to spot, or to filter for, health risks. They are also failing to *warn* of health risks.

One former diet program counselor told us, for example, that she received a phone call from a client explaining that the reason she'd missed class was that she had had her gallbladder removed. The client, whom we will call Sari, reported that her doctors had implied that her medical problem had been caused by the low-fat diet she had been on and the rapid weight loss she had experienced the past six months. This is an issue that has come up a lot with Nutri/System clients, more than 175 of whom have sued the company.

Sari asked the counselor if she thought there was a

relationship. The counselor told her that it is a possibility for anyone with a family history of gallbladder problems when they go on a low-fat diet.

The interesting thing about the conversation is that the client wasn't particularly angry about what had happened to her. She was not berating the diet company because she nearly lost her life when the gallstone dropped into her pancreas. She was simply upset that she had not been warned of the health risks. She was upset that she was not in the hands of professionals—which is what she thought the people in the white lab coats were—who would ask the right medical questions.

In our opinion, she had a right to be upset.

> *What we have in the weight loss industry is a culture of food sale, not a culture of care.*
>
> DR. ROBERT HOERR

We discovered, further, that most of the people being presented as counselors in the diet centers have no training in dealing with emotional and psychological stresses. In fact, they ordinarily don't even have nutritional backgrounds beyond their employee training by the diet center—which is less extensive and intensive than the training at Whopper College. "I don't know why those people are wearing white coats," said one client. "If you talk to them for two minutes, you know they don't have any medical background. I asked the woman who weighed me, the counselor, about setpoint, and she really didn't know what I was talking about." Another client complained that her counselor did not know anything about dietary exchanges.

Nutri/System has had the best reputation in this area. Unlike the other centers, it makes a distinction between sales personnel and counseling or service staff, even though counselors are often pressed into sales.

Now, at this diet program—considered *the leader in the field*—nutritional counselors are required to have only nine hours' worth of nutritional courses in college. Behavioral counselors must have had the same amount of coursework in psychology, social work, or some other related courses.

That's what qualifies you. Nine hours of course work. It makes no difference if the behavioral counselor's courses were Intro to Psych, Child Psych, and Art Therapy. Nine hours is nine hours.

In 1991, because of economically tight times, the company instituted what it calls cross-training. People whose nine hours' worth of nutrition classes have qualified them to be nutritional counselors now may fill in as behavioral counselors and vice versa. That means that the psychological and emotional aspect of your weight loss program may be in the hands of someone whose qualifications consist of three classes in the four basic food groups.

And this is at the program with *by far* the strictest requirement among the diet programs we investigated.

The customers of diet centers other than Nutri/System are, frequently, putting their health and weight in the hands of a high school graduate who has taken classes at the center and sat in on some sessions with customers. A great deal of the counselors' training will have covered selling the program, keeping a customer in the program, and selling the program's food. And the selling is based on emotional manipulation of frightened, desperate people.

How likely are people like this to spot medically dangerous situations—a real risk for many who join diet programs—and to act as advocate for the customer? How qualified are people like this to deal with a woman who says, "I don't think I'll ever have a normal meal again, much less a rational relationship with food"?

Take, for example, the case of a woman we will call Harriet. She was fortunate enough to be assigned a counselor who happened to have the kind of qualifications that others in her position do not have. The counselor, Marya, was a doctor from another country who was working for the diet program while she studied for her examinations for licensing in this country.

When Harriet came in for a Free Consultation, she was seen by both the center manager and Marya. The manager sold her an extensive program, but Harriet did not have enough money with her to pay for it. When she went home to get the money, Marya reported to the manager that the young woman should not be on the program. She was certain that Harriet, who circled *previously bulimic* on her health history sheet, still had an eating disorder. Her judgment was based on medical experience that the typical diet center counselor would not have. In this case, the manager insisted that the woman was fine now. The manager left the office and left the counselor to complete the sale.

Harriet returned to the office, money in hand. Marya gave her the information she needed to start the program, and they did the paperwork. While the counselor was talking, Harriet was nibbling on an apple. When they finished, she asked to use the bathroom while the counselor rang up the sale.

Marya went to the cash register and then waited for Harriet to return. She did return in a few minutes, red-faced and looking somewhat upset. Marya asked, "Did you just throw up?"

Harriet looked terribly humiliated and answered that she had. The counselor took a deep breath (because this could mean her job) and told Harriet she could not sell her the program.

In most diet programs, Harriet would have been interviewed by a person who was entirely untrained in the diagnosis of eating disorders and she would have been accepted into the program, with almost inevitably disastrous results. Indeed, there is little doubt that she actually went on to find another center or diet program that happily took her money, put her on a diet, and did not provide her with *any significant counseling*.

This is not an isolated example. Another "overqualified" counselor for a major diet chain told us:

> *I have witnessed some truly bizarre things working here. There was one morning, I was handed the chart of this woman who said she was taking three different medications for "nervousness and depression," as she stated on the information sheet. We are supposed to have medical approval for anyone*

on antidepressants because some of them could have fatal interactions with certain foods.

The manager insisted she had talked to the doctor and "everything was okay." The woman was coming in for her initial visit in an hour. I told her this was a problem and I didn't want to put the woman on the program until I spoke to the doctor. I was unable to reach the doctor or the woman, to tell her to hold off until I had cleared things.

This woman walked into my office about a half-hour later. It was obvious something was wrong. She was so foggy her speech was slurred. If it had been a teenager I would have probably assumed she was stoned on street drugs. I started to take her health history, which included attempted suicides, severe chronic depression, and so forth. She took two powerful antidepressants and a tranquilizer.

I excused myself and went to the manager's office. I told the manager it would be dangerous for the client to start without clear written and verbal permission. I could see I was getting nowhere. The manager was preoccupied with counting the food stock. She waved me off by saying the nurse was in the office; just give her a call to verify approval.

At this point I grabbed her by the arm to get her attention. "Jeanne, this woman is in bad shape, even if it were not an issue of her medications, she does not belong on the program." Jeanne was still resisting. So finally I said flat out, "Our food mixed with her drugs could kill her. Do you want that on your head? I don't!" The client was eventually sent home, and I don't know how it ended.

One counselor, who had been an elementary school teacher, told us:

One man came in who was well over 300 pounds. He had been through Optifast twice in the past three years; he was currently trying to follow Weight Watchers and failing miserably. Because of the two

Optifast losses of about 80 pounds, and the lack of any real food, he was gaining weight like crazy. I knew the problem wasn't his fault. The last thing this man needed was another diet. When people come in who are "morbidly obese" (more than double their normal weight), I feel nervous and upset. I feel totally inadequate to really help and upset that they aren't getting help.

Trained psychological counselors are not a luxury in a weight control program.

Weight Watchers provides no counseling. There is a certain amount of support that comes from meeting once a week with other people trying to lose weight. It is this aspect of the program that probably contributes most to the reports of satisfaction, even though people seldom have any permanent weight loss. But there is no provision for monitoring health problems or emotional problems.

In the menu programs, considerably more time is spent in "counseling." At some centers, the client comes in every day and may spend an almost unlimited time with her counselor. The problem is that the counselor, again, is untrained. She knows the program. She probably lost weight on the program. But she has no training in dealing with eating disorders or the emotional problems that arise during the stress of a diet. She has no medical knowledge to help her pinpoint potential health problems. She has no nutritional knowledge. And finally, she *does not know how to help you control your weight.*

It is difficult to think that any real counseling takes place when a counselor states, as one Diet Center counselor did, that she is careful about the questions she asks of the clients. They all relate to the mechanics of adhering to the program. Otherwise, she told us, she feared she might "open up a can of worms" she wasn't equipped to handle.

EDUCATION AND BEHAVIORAL CONDITIONING

Most of the programs claim to "teach you how to eat for the rest of your life." That's an admirable objective. If you are going to manage your weight and food in the future, there is a lot you need to know. Not that you have to be able to write a Ph.D. thesis on nutrition and weight loss, but you need better information than you probably have now. So, do the diet programs deliver here?

There is less to this than meets the eye.

TALLULAH BANKHEAD

Unfortunately, they don't. On any given diet program, you will probably not learn *anything* other than what that particular program is about. You will live on liquid nutrition or have someone else give you a menu.

This lack of current, credible information and presentation is a big problem, caused primarily by the fact that classes, unlike food, don't generate revenue. Most diet center staff people don't know enough to teach you. Occasionally, staff people are employed who have more expertise, but they are allowed to give you only the information approved by the company. More information might take the shine off the mystique of the diet or diet food they are selling. In fact, a behavioral counselor will be rebuked for not following the class manual exactly. Even changing the order of the topics presented at the class meetings is frowned on. In other words, no matter what is bothering the class members that day, they may have to suffer through a lecture on "improved grocery shopping."

This was a major criticism in every evaluation of the programs we looked at. In fact, the staff and clients we interviewed describe the classes offered as boring, worthless, or an outright, irritating insult. They said the kind of information offered was available in any newsstand magazine, the kind that offer suggestions on "Trim Thighs in Twenty Days" side by side with articles on how to "Seduce Your Family with Sinful Chocolate Desserts."

"A counselor with no more background in the subject of weight control than I have," said one Nutri/System client, "read to us from the company manual." A Jenny Craig client reported that the educational component of that program consisted of watching movies of Jenny lecturing on different subjects, movies that almost no one attended.

There were many clients who complained that they could not get information when they specifically asked for it. "When I asked why I had to limit my vegetable intake to three half-cup servings, or why I had to have my snack two hours after lunch, or why I couldn't substitute a certain candy for a fat/carbohydrate exchange, or why whole grain bread and cereals were not allowed, I always got the same pat answer: 'that is how the program is designed,' or 'that's how we feel you will lose weight the quickest.' No explanation of why. I don't think anybody really knew why!"

Another client described how a counselor disobeyed the company policy by allowing her to look at the food nutrient list. "I asked to see the calories and fat in some of the foods I ordered. I wanted to know if there were differences in what I was eating. I wanted a little control over my own fate. With this information I could compare the food to the things I see in the grocery store. I thought it would give me an idea of how to do this on my own, even how to feed my family better. At first she was reluctant. She said the list was only for the counselor's use. In the end, she did make a copy and give it to me the following week. She told me to fold it away carefully in my purse so that no one would see it."

Most diet programs now recognize all the studies that have been done on the metabolism of fat versus carbohydrate. Almost all programs incorporate the low-fat approach in their diets. But in terms of client education, none is offered. If you ask the average client why she is on a low-fat prepackaged food program, she will reply that it is "less fattening." She has not been told anything else.

As for behavioral conditioning, no one knows how and to what extent it really works. In the major study done in this area, the eating habits of the subjects were changed and they lost weight. However, the weight loss may simply have resulted from the *fact* of, not the nature of, the changes. The changes certainly did not mimic the eating habits of "natural thins," as most of the diet centers now suggest. In addition, studies done since 1985 about the long-range impact of behavioral conditioning have changed professional thinking on this point. What psychologists once thought was the "magic bullet" for dieters did not change the final outcome. Dieters have about the same track record after two years, with or without behavioral conditioning.

Presented as gospel in most of the behavioral conditioning sessions are such rules as "Never eat standing up," "Never do anything else while you're eating, except talk to another person," "Never shop when you're hungry." Most people who have read as many as three women's magazines a year in the last ten years could fill out the rest of the list. There is no medical or scientific basis for any of these rules. One counselor who has herself successfully controlled her weight for years—*not* by using her company's program—said she couldn't imagine eating alone without reading. Another said she often shopped when she was hungry because then even the healthiest foods looked good. This "behavioral conditioning" is approximately as sophisticated as makeup tips.

The classes are so useless that most clients stop attending very quickly, and some centers have discontinued them.

EXERCISE PROGRAMS

When most of the diet centers first opened their doors, the link between exercise and weight had not been as clearly established as it is now. However, in the last decade of the twentieth century, the connection is unchallenged. Without exercise, weight loss is an uphill battle. And if you reach the top of the hill, you tumble down with great rapidity.

Since it became clear to the medical and scientific communities that the only road to long-term weight loss includes exercise, the diet centers have started paying lip service. But they might as well be ventriloquists. Nutri/System, for example, offers two exercise videotapes (at an extra charge, as we pointed out) and asks the customer if she's using them. The Jenny Craig exercise audio tape is part of an expensive supplementary package. Weight Watchers outlines a program of activities and asks the customer if she's using it. Most of the others just *tell* their clients they really ought to get some exercise.

6

Unqualified, Unregulated, and Unlikely to Change

ㄷ—ㄲ

> *There are people in this program I know*
> *are bulimic. The management will sell*
> *the program to anyone with the money.*

DIET PROGRAM COUNSELOR

ONE MAJOR OBJECTION we have to the diet centers is that they are a business, and that is not appropriate for such an important health issue.

Weight, dieting, and the health problems that dieting can cause are potentially a great deal more dangerous than problems with your teeth, feet, skin, or even your eyes. And yet dentists, podiatrists, dermatologists, and both ophthalmologists and optometrists are trained and licensed professionals. The persons who enlist you in a diet program and guide you through it are salesmen. (We know that we should use the less sexist term *salespeople,* but right now we want the old word and all its associations.) Many of the abuses we found in the diet system arise directly out of an unacceptably close relationship between decision making and profit making.

SELLING THE PROGRAM

The liquid fasting programs *insert* business procedures and profit making into a professional medical situation. Because they are so often paid for by health insurance, there is no need for a hard-sell approach. A patient is referred to Optifast, Medifast, or Health Management Resources by a doctor, often the doctor out of whose office the program is being administered. Each patient (or his or her health insurance company) pays about $500 a month for sometimes as long as ten or twelve months. About 75 percent of that goes for expenses, including the doctor's fees. The other 25 percent is *profit* for the hospital or doctor's office.

Representative Ron Wyden, in his investigation of the diet industry, discovered a Medifast "income prospectus" that told doctors they could take in $22,000 net in a year by treating just twenty patients. Remember, the treatment includes *one* examination by the doctor.

"Here's what I got for $2,000," says Georgia, a former Optifast patient. "A fifteen-minute medical exam, weigh-in, blood work, the routine stuff. Every week a nurse weighed me, took blood every other week, and gave me a pep talk, depending on how the scale looked. I went to these weekly classes for a while. They were really dumb. The leader had less training in psychology than me, and he harped each week about our being in denial . . . I have grown to hate that word."

The question then is this. Should doctors be prescribing for their patients programs that do not work, that are enormously costly to health insurance companies, and from which the doctors, or their colleagues, reap significant profits?

In the food-inclusive and menu programs, a lot of the business-related abuses occur during the Free Consultation, which is the diet center's most powerful sales tool.

Most of us know to what lengths salespeople will go to get a potential customer onto their turf. Land developers, for example, offer premiums to get you to come to a hotel conference room and watch a slide show. The diet centers advertise "special offers" . . . and withhold information. If you want to know what the program is and what it costs, you have to sit down across the desk from a salesperson with a hell of a lot more training in sales methods than your nutritional counselor will have in nutrition. Many of the worst problems in the diet programs come up because these people are under pressure to sell. (This is, of course, not true of noncommercial groups such as TOPS.)

> *I would rather be the man who bought the Brooklyn Bridge than the man who sold it.*
>
> WILL ROGERS

Many people who call or come into a diet center are ready to buy. They are desperate and frightened and feel they do not have any other alternative. Human misery is easy to appeal to, and society has made these people pretty miserable. In that sort of case, the Free Consultation is just a matter of determining how expensive a program this unhappy individual will sign up for. (Even if this is the third or fourth diet program for the client, she is not usually irate at having to start all over. There is a kind of passive acceptance of the idea that she is to blame for her failure to follow through, to keep the weight off.) It is the first-timers, and those who have not already made up their minds to buy the program, who offer the salesperson real scope.

The average potential client is a woman. There are male clients, but they are few and far between. This woman is between the ages of thirty-five and fifty, a competent professional or a responsible wife and mother, or both. Over a number of years of trying to mold her body into a shape that is more acceptable to contemporary American aesthetic standards, she has come to measure her self-worth by the numbers on the scale. She has tried at least one other diet center, and her self-esteem has been further eroded by that experience. She views her failure to lose weight as a sign of her own weakness and moral inadequacy. And she has been encouraged in this view by those around her, including the diet center that did not live up to its claim to be able to help her.

She is not considering another diet program casually.

She is not there just to lose an extra ten pounds before her sister's wedding. She could be described as having a subclinical eating disorder, or is well on her way. Because of her relationship with food and eating, she is less than healthy and lacks energy and a reliable immune system. She may be amenorrheic entirely or have menstrual periods very irregularly. But her physical condition is not nearly so impaired as her emotional and mental state. This is how she describes herself and her life:

> My body is my worst enemy. The second I am not on guard it betrays me. I never trust myself. I haven't the least idea of whether I'm hungry or not. In fact, I almost never eat when I'm hungry. I eat when I feel vulnerable, which is almost always because I am fat.
>
> I know the way the day will go when I weigh myself in the morning. Sometimes I keep on weighing myself all day long.
>
> I wake up thinking it's going to be okay. I've got a terrific family, and my writing is really starting to take shape. And then I weigh myself, and it's all over.
>
> I can't eat with my family anymore. Their food is too fattening.
>
> I can't shop for groceries or cook. I have my husband and kids do it. I just can't be around food. I'm terrified of being caught in the grocery store as I break open bags of food, eat a handful and then toss them away.
>
> Can you imagine? Breast cancer, surgery, chemotherapy . . . and I still can't lose weight. I'm so depressed. I'll never lose this ten pounds.

This woman, upon walking into a liquid fasting, food-inclusive, or menu program diet center, will find herself sitting with an interested, sympathetic person. At Nutri/

System, this will probably be someone who does only sales, although nutritional and behavioral counselors do get recruited. At Jenny Craig, only the manager is trusted to make sales. This counselor/salesperson asks concerned questions to discover what is really bothering the potential client about her weight.

Is she afraid she won't get promoted at work? Does she think her husband is starting to be disgusted with the way she looks? Are her children making her feel that they're embarrassed? The salesperson keeps asking until she finds the customer's greatest concern. From then on, that issue will come up again and again, especially if the customer seems to think the cost is too high or wonders about the time involved or thinks she might go talk to the competition first. In the training workshops of at least one diet center, this is called the "hot spot."

The hot spot. A woman's deepest fear. Find it and use it and you've just sold another contract.

At the diet centers, these are the basic sales techniques:

- raise hopes
- inspire confidence in your own expertise
- build trust and/or dependence
- target fears and weaknesses

The counselor/salesperson may refer to herself as a model of weight loss. (She has been hired for her resemblance to the tall and slender media role models.) She may have the temerity to tell the client she was once much bigger and that she too lost weight on the program, even if it isn't true. Many of the salespeople in the fasting and food-inclusive programs haven't the vaguest idea of what it feels like to go on a diet. (There is a different situation in menu programs and support groups.)

Or she may start by showing the pictures on the wall of success stories, clients who lost many pounds on the program. There are before and after pictures to document the success. Of course, no one mentions to the prospective client that the "after" picture was taken the day the client hit her goal weight. Who knows what she weighs six months or a year later? She may be back on the program again.

The manager or counselor will point to the pictures and say, "imagine how thrilled your husband will be when you look like that!" The conversation will continue along the lines of this one, a composite of sales pitches heard by or reported to us.

SALESPERSON: Your husband won't look at another woman again, when he sees your new body.

CLIENT: I hope so.

SALESPERSON: Have you been worried about that lately?

CLIENT: Well. He says nothing has changed.

SALESPERSON: But it doesn't feel that way to you.

CLIENT: Lately, it seems like he's avoiding me.

SALESPERSON: Sexually?

CLIENT: Yes. He says there isn't anyone else, but . . .

SALESPERSON: But he doesn't seem to want to make love to you?

CLIENT: This is pretty personal.

SALESPERSON: Don't worry. I'm just here to help.

"They sold the program," said one former Jenny Craig client, "like they were doing some kind of humanitarian work. There was such empathy and concern in the beginning. It didn't stay that way when I stopped losing. When I finally quit coming, no one ever called to see if I was okay."

SALESPERSON: Robert got a major promotion after he lost the fifty pounds. He really showed the company the kind of willpower and character he has.

CLIENT: That would be great.

SALESPERSON: So much of it's just a matter of confidence.

CLIENT: I really need that kind of confidence. I know people look at me like I'm lazy and undisciplined.

SALESPERSON: That can really hold you back, you know.

CLIENT: Yeah, I know.

SALESPERSON: It's the image you present to your co-workers and your boss. It's really important.

CLIENT: I know. I could never ask for a raise without losing weight.

Being indolent, lazy, and out of control may be a far cry from the truth for the average overweight person. But the diet program's sales staff uses it nonetheless. With the client's low opinion of herself, you could probably sell her a gold bracelet guaranteed to take off weight as long as she wears it. If the only way to gain self-esteem is to lose weight, you simply convince the customer that you are going to do that for her. All she has to do is show up.

SALESPERSON: Glenda was so shy when she started the program, she barely spoke to people. Now she is in all kinds of groups and is always out with friends. She's a real social butterfly.

CLIENT: That sounds like paradise.

SALESPERSON: That sort of thing is difficult for you?

CLIENT: Well . . .

SALESPERSON: Lots of people are shy, especially when they don't feel that they look their best. And, of course, there are the vibrations you pick up from other people.

CLIENT: No matter where I go, I don't seem to belong. Right now I wouldn't even go with friends where I could meet people. I'm just grossed out by my appearance. What man would talk to me anyway?

SALESPERSON: That all changed for Glenda. I'm sure it can change for you.

And then there is flattery. "I can't believe you have two grownup children, you look so young." "You must have been a dancer when you were young; you have perfectly shaped legs" (to a woman who is concerned about her expanding waistline). "A few pounds is going to make all the difference for a woman with such a lovely face." "A grandmother? No! I don't believe it!"

It's a business.

She can, of course, combine flattery and fear, flattery and hope, fear and trust—the possibilities are endless. Once she can establish a psychological hook, she has the makings of a sale. For instance, the consultant will ask what size dress you once wore. Then, "An eight, that's wonderful! Remember what it felt like to go into a store and put on a size eight and look great in it," she says. Even if the last time you saw a size eight was in high school.

> One may smile, and smile, and be a
> villain.

> WILLIAM SHAKESPEARE

Or, "You want to lose weight for your wedding. That's terrific! I can imagine how unhappy this extra weight makes you. I understand why you wouldn't shop for a wedding dress now. But think of what you'll look like in three months."

"You're right," she agrees, "extra weight definitely makes a woman look and feel older. Luckily you have such a youthful face, a few pounds will make you look like a teen again."

On and on it goes. If you hesitate because of price, the counselor reminds you "you owe it to yourself" to do this. After all, isn't this the reason you are overweight to begin with, that you haven't taken care of yourself?

And, of course, this manipulation is particularly effective in a society that has, in the past few decades, begun to treat weight as a moral issue. Fat people are seen as undisciplined, lacking in character, probably emotionally disturbed. This message is reinforced by everything from advertising to the well-meant advice of aunts and uncles.

"Fat people" jokes are just about the only form of personally denigrating humor still allowable in the media. Women, ethnic minorities, and even mothers-in-law are now, to some degree, protected from gross insult. People who weigh more than 20 percent above the national average are not.

A diet center salesperson need only play on a plethora of already highly developed negative feelings. Throughout the sales pitch, the classes, and the counseling, a customer's emotions—fear, guilt, self-loathing—are used and fostered to keep her money coming into the program. Exploitation doesn't get much more rank than this. In the end, then, the diet centers turn out people who are not only physically more prone to fat than when they entered but emotionally more vulnerable as well.

The connection between the size and shape of your body and your feelings of self-esteem is, in large part, what allows the diet con game to succeed. Program advertising and sales hype play on making you feel inadequate. They are ready to sell you the answer to your inadequacies, and, while they are at it, they will address your long-standing neuroses. They sell the program with their "empathy" and willingness to take on all your problem behavior, your obsessive-compulsive or emotional attachment to food. They are going to cure it all . . . with a staff that has been trained at Diet Program Central for a week.

But, if other training is minimal, sales training is intensive. For weeks the novice management trainee learns how to deal with every type of client, to present "information" in a positive light, without really giving any information at all. These are not people with training in psychology, human services, or social work, but they are drilled in all the vulnerable emotional areas for a potential client. Whether you use the phrase "hot spot," as the program mentioned earlier in the chapter does, or simply turn the consultation into a tear-jerking melodrama, the result is the same. You've made another sale.

At most centers, everybody on the staff ends up selling something. The receptionist pushes extra food supplements. The "counselors" keep you strictly adhering to the prescribed diet so that you have to buy all your food from the center. At Jenny Craig, your counselor's take-home pay is based on food sales.

One counselor from a nationwide chain reported to us a gross example of manipulation to make a program sale. The prospective client, whom we'll call Kelly, was a very emotional and very depressed woman whose mother had recently died. Her stress was still very apparent in tearful bouts during the sales consultation. Her state over the past few months had already had an impact on her physically as well. Following her mother's death she developed a medical problem which was treated with cortisone drugs. Such drugs are notorious for producing bloating and rapid weight gain.

Kelly already suffered from debilitating eating behavior, ranging from fasting to diet pills. In fact, the counselor who reported to us was able to describe her as having a subclinical eating disorder after their first few meetings.

At Kelly's Free Consultation, the salesperson confronted a "potential customer" who was grieving, was in physical and emotional pain, and was twenty pounds heavier than she had been six months before. She described herself as panicked. Her eating was completely out of control.

Kelly was comforted and counseled by the salesperson, who assured the distraught woman that the program was the answer to her problems. The diet program would "fix" everything from her grief over the loss of her mother to the damage done by the cortisone drug. When the salesperson was unable to console the client completely or assuage her fears, the center's behavioral counselor was called into the consultation as backup. Again the client was led to believe, by virtue of the behavioral counselor's presence, that she was in competent hands, that whatever her problem was, the program was equipped to deal with it.

I never wonder to see men wicked, but I
often wonder to see them not ashamed.

JONATHAN SWIFT

Kelly was sold the most expensive lifetime program. She stayed in the program about five weeks. The first two weeks, eating about half of the packaged food, she lost two and a half pounds. In the next three weeks she gained it back plus two more pounds. She could not battle with the program requirements and with her own sense of failure and worthlessness and she dropped out.

And just who are these people who are willing to sell a grieving woman just out of cortisone treatment and with a history of eating disorders an expensive program she is unable to stay on for a month? Who are these people who are selling to anyone who walks in the door the American dream of being young, *slim*, and beautiful?

Well, those are the job qualifications—being young, slim, and beautiful.

Never mind if your only job since high school was managing a Toys R Us store. If you look like the image and can learn the company line, you're in. Of the diet program staff we surveyed, only three people had an educational background that was in any way related to their work. Many admitted that one of the problems of the program is that the staff was not able to handle the level of emotional, and in some cases physical, problems presented by clients. This might even be acceptable for sales, if there were any professional backup for client evaluation. In most centers, however, the salesperson is also the counselor.

And you move up in the company, not by being a wise, informed, and sympathetic counselor, but by being tall, blond, and willowy and having a hard-nosed knack for sales.

However, before you start to think that we are saying this con game works because all of these nice women are really blood-sucking slimeballs or clever charlatans, let us point out that that is not always the case. There are some reasonably nice people in the diet programs who simply *don't know what they're talking about*. This is especially true for those who have "come up through the system."

Answers to our interview questions confirmed that the naïveté of the counselor often works to the company's advantage in sales. The less she really knows, the more enthusiastically and sincerely she will sell the program. The same counselors who said almost all the clients regained the weight they lost did not understand why diets were not a viable way to deal with overweight (or perceived overweight). One counselor we interviewed agreed that most clients gain back all the weight they lose and admitted she didn't know why. She assumed "they just started eating all the wrong things again." When these counselors were asked if they had read (or were familiar with) six of the most recognized current weight loss books, the answers were an overwhelming no. Only about a quarter of those interviewed had heard of *any* of the books.

This is an important piece of the puzzle. Our interviews revealed that not only are most of the counseling staff of diet centers limited in their knowledge of weight loss to company training, information, and biases, a great many, in programs like Jenny Craig, Diet Center, and Weight Watchers, are graduates of the program themselves. That means they successfully completed the program and were then trained as counselor/salespersons or group leaders. They have experienced success themselves and, *by continuing to stay connected to the program,* this very small minority usually manages to keep their weight off.

Gretchen is a good example of this sort of counselor. She worked for some time at one of the diet programs where staff are former clients. While there, she had kept her weight down. When her office closed, she immediately began to gain weight. *But she still believed.* She did not recognize that the only reason for her success—as opposed to the failure of the overwhelming majority of her clients—was that the program had become her life.

So Gretchen went to another major diet program to enroll, explaining to the salesperson that she had "failed to follow the rules" after she lost her job.

Gretchen and the others like her are the sincerest, most believable salespeople possible. At the level of the local center or group, many of the company employees still believe the program is a good thing, in spite of their expe-

rience with client dropout and the magnitude of the regaining weight problem.

For instance, in the support group type, where successful program participation is mandatory for leaders, there
was much less cynicism. These people said they would
recommend the program to a friend, and they were more
cautious and less critical of the program when asked why
most people gained the weight back. Although the facts
didn't add up, *although they watched the vast majority of
people fail on the program*, they were reluctant to condemn it.

> *Great evil has been done on earth by peo-
> ple who think they have all the answers.*
>
> RUBY PLENTY CHIEFS

On the surface this doesn't make sense. But it makes
very good sales sense. Who better than a convert to sell
the program? Who will have more missionary zeal than
someone who has been successful on the program? She
may even honestly believe that, if others put in her hard
work and commitment, they could also succeed. She is
living proof of the dream.

As for those who did not come up through the program,
many of them are sincere, too . . . until they quit. Many of
the counselors we interviewed were drawn to working with
the diet programs because they saw the work as service
to others. They wanted to help people. If they had not
experienced serious weight or eating problems themselves,
they believed what they were taught in training. It was
only after they had worked in the programs themselves
that these counselors realized how useless the programs
were. And then they found other jobs.

> *Our worst enemies here are not the igno-
> rant and the simple, however cruel; our*

> *worst enemies are the intelligent and
> the corrupt.*
>
> GRAHAM GREENE

ABUSES

The more reputable diet centers have claimed that they take pains not to sell the program to unsuitable clients. Nutri/System, in particular, has company policies against sales in medically inadvisable situations.

However, we have been told by the staff of various programs that this aspect of quality has diminished as the economy has worsened. A few years ago, because the diet programs were overflowing, revenue was excellent and the staff more professional, restrictions in diet programs were more tightly monitored. If someone came in with complicating medical problems, that person might not be sold the program.

In most branches of the big diet programs, now, anyone with the money to buy the program can buy the program, including people with diabetes or hypertension, people on a variety of antidepressants and tranquilizers, and people with clear eating disorders. Company policy can be circumvented in order to bolster flagging sales.

What makes this possible, what lets the company off the hook, is that there is no requirement for a physical exam before starting the program. The client is the one who makes the assessment of her health status in the form of a simple "health history profile." If the prospective client states that she does not have diabetes, the salesperson is satisfied that she does not have diabetes. And, since it would jeopardize a program sale to believe otherwise, she does not make too much of questionable responses. And, of course, clients do lie. Often, their doctors have warned them against entering a program and they know they will not get his or her approval, which will be required of them if they admit to a health problem.

The simple requirement of a letter of approval from the client's doctor is another way around the problem. These letters of approval are not verified by the center and there is no requirement that they refer specifically to the condition in the client's medical history which has raised the question of suitability. A note on a doctor's letterhead saying, "Mary Jones can be on a diet program" is all that is required. As long as that letter is in the file, the client can begin the program. Mary Jones might have gotten the letter from a doctor who knows nothing about her antidepressants, or one who has no knowledge of her history of eating disorders, but the letter presumably relieves the diet center of responsibility.

Also, the counselor we quoted earlier is not the only one to be "nervous and upset" about morbidly obese people in diet centers. Their presence there is, at best, useless. (Imagine a 375-pound person being helped by Diet Center.) At worst, it is jeopardizing the client's life by adding still more weight. In an effort to protect themselves, some programs—a very few—have put restrictions on the amount of weight to be lost. If projected weight loss is above a certain amount, a doctor's consent is required.

This presents a problem for the sales staff. Most clients, of course, don't want to spend money to go to the doctor to be weighed and scolded, especially if they think there is some magic in the food or supplements that the doctor would not approve. So the diet center's sales staff knows that, if they send the client off to get permission, she probably won't come back. Well, every manager knows there are ways to get around this and get the sale. Here's how they work it.

Say the rule is that, if a client has a hundred pounds to lose, she needs to see her doctor. The salesperson tells her that, in order to avoid that hassle, her "first" goal will be set at sixty pounds. Later, she can sign another contract for the next forty. Presto! No doctor.

Another counselor we interviewed reported pressure from the management of her center to ignore her program's medical policies. She was a psychologist whose training in eating disorders often brought her head to head with her managers. Remember as you read her story that

her job might just as easily have been filled by someone
with no training in psychology at all.

*A new client is starting the program. As a nutri-
tional counselor, I am given her chart to assess.
Unfortunately, it's only a minute before the client
walks into my office and so there is little to do if
there is any problem with her beginning the program
this evening except apologize and send her home.*

*The first and most critical part of the new client
assessment is to review the client's health history
form. My company policy states there are more than
a dozen conditions that require a doctor's approval
before admitting a client to the program. This means
both written and verbal in the case of diabetes or
hypertension. It also includes clients who have been
anorexic or bulimic. At one time, they were not admitted at all. If in treatment, they must also have
the approval of a therapist.*

*I note the client has circled bulimia [on the form].
I call it to the attention of my immediate supervisor,
who is in the office observing. His response is why
don't I simply ask the client how long ago any inci-
dence of bulimia occurred. Also, he is under the
impression that "the client does not really throw up.
She 'only' uses laxatives and diuretics."*

*I see the client. She confirms the problem is re-
cent. In the past she did use vomiting to purge. However, currently she limits herself to laxatives. I ask
if she is under treatment for eating disorders. To
which she responds no, she has never been diagnosed as such. But she has also never gone to a
doctor about the problem, hence the lack of
diagnosis.*

*I leave the room and approach my supervisor and
actually break in on a meeting with the manager of
the entire city. "We have a problem here, [I say].
The woman in my office has a significant eating disorder. I will not take responsibility for seeing her."*

*I detail the client's responses. "If either of you wish
to treat her, I cannot stop you."*

*Sensing my anger and resolve on this issue, both
managers assure me that they had no previous
knowledge of the problem. And, since the young
woman was never "diagnosed" with an eating disorder, there was no problem with her starting the
program. I state that as an eating disorder counselor, I have an ethical problem in seeing her. And
after this evening they will have to assign a different
nutritional counselor to the client.*

*After the shift ends, when I speak to the office
manager, he lets me know in a way how this will be
handled. They will simply have this "undiagnosed"
client fill out a new health history form. The original
problem will never show up.*

*I respond, "I plan to check that chart every week
and if anything is changed I'll write a letter to the
president of the company with a copy to the local
newspaper."*

This kind of abuse, of course, is not officially sanctioned
by the national offices. Indeed, it is a violation of company
policy. At the same time, success on the job is measured
not in customer satisfaction but in dollars taken in. You
don't take in dollars by turning away customers.

Again and again, we see the danger of having a health-
oriented industry being run without regulations and with
a strong profit orientation. The national office can institute
policies that, if properly enforced, would provide a certain
amount of protection against client abuse. However, so
long as the incomes of the staff depend on sales, there
will be people who manage to get around those policies.

One Nutri/System counselor reported that her center
manager would charge in on Friday and say, "All right,
girls. We need three upsells today or I don't pay my rent."
(Upsells are sales of more expensive programs to people
who come in to take advantage of a special offer. In other
words, bait and switch.)

The reason this woman needed the sales to pay her rent

was that she is paid minimum wage plus commission. In other words, the person who is in charge of the entire center, the one who does the hiring and firing and scheduling of workers, makes no more than a busboy unless she can sell, sell, sell. Her income depends on sales, and she has the power to affect the incomes of the people working under her.

Indiscriminate sales of the program to people who should not be on it is, therefore, an abuse built into the system.

Another problem is the sale of programs to already slender people. One counselor stated how surprised she was to see that there were so many women her size on the program, some smaller. She had always thought of herself as average.

Joe, a Jenny Craig client's husband, commented to us, "I never expected to see so many normal-looking women in a diet center. I would sit in the lobby waiting for my wife, thinking that all these women must be at the end of the program; the only other possibility is they have something wrong with their heads."

"I was shocked," said one former counselor. "I looked at the client's chart before she started the program. She was five two and weighed 108 pounds. The computer said her weight range was 104 to 114, so they sold her a program to lose 4 pounds. Imagine! There is something wrong with that woman and it's not her weight."

It will probably cost her $400 to lose that 4 pounds.

And there probably is something wrong with her head, so to speak. A woman who is five two and weighs 108 and is so convinced she is fat that she is willing to pay money to lose weight is, at the very least, suffering from a severely distorted perception of her body image, which is one important warning sign of an eating disorder. It's irresponsible, at best, to encourage her delusions.

There are also branches of diet centers in poor communities, in which Free Consultations are given to women on welfare who are then sold the program, even if all they can afford is a special $39.95 four-week offer and they have sixty pounds or more to lose.

THE BOTTOM LINE

In most states, diet centers are not considered medical programs and therefore are not regulated. The major diet programs do have policies about the more serious health issues, and they insist that self-regulation is enough. It isn't.

"In June 1990," according to *The New York Times*, "the New York City Department of Consumer Affairs reported the following based on undercover visits by its staff: nine out of ten diet programs in New York City fail to warn potential customers of health risks associated with rapid weight loss; others engage in quackery and pressure thin people to sign up for costly programs."

In March of 1993, the National Institutes of Health released the results of a full-scale investigation of the current state of the diet industry. One of the outcomes was that the Federal Trade Commission has signed what one official called an "out-of-court agreement" with three major diet programs to change their advertising claims, claims that imply "long-term weight loss" and "cure."

The diet programs were born in the last couple of decades and, with any luck and some good legislation, they will die during this one. They are selling hope. People want to believe that this time it will happen. They are selling respectability. If you think you are overweight, dieting is the socially correct thing to do. They are selling happiness. Happiness, Charlie Brown, is a thin bottom.

They are selling love, sexuality, self-esteem, social grace, and charm. They are promising Mr. Right, status, class, success, job promotions, marital bliss, glamour, and a dozen other things. All the things that a beautiful figure can buy. All the things we, especially women, think are dependent on the size and shape of our bodies.

None of the above-mentioned program extras is actually highlighted in the sales contract. But they certainly are worked over in the sales approach. They are the client/company silent understanding. It's what they offer you for the low, low price of $19.95.

But they can't deliver.

PART II
What Will Work For You

If you have built castles in the air, your work need not be lost; that is where they should be. Now put foundations under them.

HENRY DAVID THOREAU

7

Designing Your Own Program or, Resetting Your Setpoint, Reclaiming Your Life

◦━━▸

*I know as much as the [diet center] coun-
selors. I just don't know how to get myself to do it.*

DIET PROGRAM CLIENT

THERE ARE THREE basic principles of effective weight control, all of which are violated blatantly and grossly by the
program diet centers and, to some degree, by all organized
weight control groups. They should serve as the structure
for designing your own program. If you adopt these principles and develop the skills to implement them in your life,
everything else, such as calories and portion size, will fall
into place.

TAKING CONTROL

*My mother put me on my first diet when
I was twelve. I've been through fifteen
years of everyone telling me when and
what to eat. I've reached the point that*

77

*I'm burnt out, but if I stop I'll blow up
like a balloon.*

DIET PROGRAM CLIENT

Developing a lasting, healthy relationship with food and
your body involves taking control, the exact opposite of
what happens when you go to a diet center.

Belief in magic has always been the refuge of those
who feel powerless. The illusion of magic in dieting keeps
the dieter in a powerless position. And it is only one short
step from powerless to hopeless. In buying into the miracle
cure, the individual loses sight of any real impact she
might have on the problem. "I've been doing this since I
was twelve," says Loretta, a former Nutri/System client.
"I'm in my forties, and you'd think by now I'd get it
straight. As long as I'm on the diet 100 percent, I'm okay.
The first bag of chips and it's the end."

When a mature, intelligent woman can be defeated totally by one bag of chips—or even a new bakery down
the street—something's wrong. If she were making her
own decisions about food, eating those chips would not
be "getting out of control." It would be deciding to use
part of her "fat budget" on something frivolous, and it
would carry no more emotional weight than buying a pair
of ten-dollar earrings that she didn't really need.

There are few differences in attitude greater than that
between *self-control* and *taking control*. The former are
words that people who don't fit the currently fashionable
slim silhouette hear all the time. "Don't you have any
self-control?" "All you need is a little self-control." "If
you don't have enough self-control to get your weight
down, why should we think you can . . ." Run an office.
Stick with a project. Finish a course. You fill in the
blank yourself.

*Somewhere deep down inside we know
that in the final analysis we do decide
things and that even our decisions to let*

*someone else decide are really our deci-
sions, however pusillanimous.*

HARVEY COX

So you try to cultivate self-control. But that, unfortunately, doesn't mean putting your "self" in the driver's
seat. It almost always means trying to get your "self" to
meet demands from outside, to fit other people's patterns
and meet other people's expectations. It means developing
the iron will to do what every fiber of your being is telling
you not to do, and to do it because someone else thinks
it's best for you.

Consider how passive you are at Nutri/System or Jenny
Craig. You are told exactly when, what, and how much
to eat. In most instances, your only active participation is
stepping on the scale for a weigh-in. And then, as often
as not, what little sense of independence you manage to
maintain is undermined by a punitive counselor who
scolds you for breaking the rules. One result is that you
become reliant on the diet system. Another is that self-
control and self-respect become synonymous. The same
thing can happen to you from just living and breathing the
"diet air" of our culture. If you read magazines, listen to
your friends, and watch television, you absorb the diet
mentality.

Giving in to what you like and want creates self-
loathing. Your preferences, cravings, joys, and needs—the
things that make up your personality—all become the
enemy.

You have to get out of that mentality. Until you do,
you can't create your own way of eating and moving. You
won't even know what's important to you and what isn't.

However, most longtime dieters, when you talk about
just abandoning dieting cold turkey, are terrified. You can
see the look of fear in their eyes. "You must be crazy,"
they say. "In a couple of months I won't fit through the
door. If I'm not on a diet I'm completely out of control.
If I just eat what I want, I'll go wild with food." Most
of us who are restricted eaters have spent so much of our

lives controlling ourselves we are terrified to make the enormous leap of faith required. The structures and eating guidelines of Weight Watchers or the Rotation Diet or even some nebulous idea of "good eating" have become our life jacket in a sea of impulse eating and emotional hunger. Even if we get the courage to try eating whenever and whatever we want, the first breakdown in the plan causes us to rush back to dieting, with the built-in security of its rules.

Of course, only a handful of people can eat by the rules forever, and they are usually the same people who always color in the lines and think toothbrushes are floor-cleaning tools. The rest of us need to break free. We know the life jacket is really a straitjacket and we need to shed it. But we're not quite ready to stand around naked.

So, how do lifelong dieters find needed security without simply creating another diet? That's where *taking* control comes in.

In the area of weight, control is a major issue. Many weight problems and eating disorders have at their core a lack of control over important life issues. Controlling food is a symbolic way to control life. Many people with weight problems come from families where there are strict controls over attitude and behavior. With the best intentions in the world, parents in these families rear their children to meet the parents' own standards and expectations and leave little room for individual choices. This usually begins with issues of morality, where it may be positive and important, and spreads to issues of taste, such as hairstyles and clothing choices, where it can be oppressive.

Indeed, in this society, most women face that kind of outside control from all sides. The limits of acceptable behavior for women are very narrow. Food, being one of the few things over which the individual herself has control, often becomes an area of self-expression. And, since it is critical that people have freedom and self-expression in their lives, overeating can actually be a way of maintaining emotional health.

However, this way of using food to rebel against the structures others create for us has obvious drawbacks. It is not, in the end, the healthiest solution to the problem. Taking control in a more positive sense starts with recognizing this fact and separating food from the *symbolism* of food.

> *Abstainer, n. A weak person who yields to the temptation of denying himself a pleasure.*

> AMBROSE BIERCE

In other words, instead of robbing yourself of one important area in which you are free—as the diet programs do—we are suggesting that you make yourself free in other ways, that you exercise control in a healthier, stronger way. We are suggesting that you take control of your life and environment rather than trying to control yourself.

Taking control means rejecting out of hand the structures created for you by others and starting from scratch with the person you are. It means making your environment adjust to you instead of adjusting to your environment. It means believing that you have the intelligence and ability to evaluate your situation and make decisions.

If self-control says "Resist the desire to eat chocolate ice cream," taking control says, "Why should I? I like it. I think I'll take a look at my options." If self-control says, "There's no reason John shouldn't leave candy bars around, just because they're a temptation to me. I have to be strong," taking control says, "I don't want that Snickers in my face!"

Control, in this sense, has to go beyond just your eating environment. Indeed, it may not begin with food at all. You may need to set limits and create boundaries in your personal or professional life. If your life at home is one of constant stress, for example, you may not be able to afford to give up your eating patterns. They're serving too important a purpose in your life. Instead, you may need to begin with making small changes in what your family expects of you and what you can expect of them.

Taking control may mean imagining a life for yourself, going beyond the limits you've accepted and thinking what your life could be. We're not suggesting that you begin tomorrow by opening a school for disadvantaged children in your living room, but maybe you could begin by reading about Marva Collins, who did just that, as a way to remind yourself of the possibilities of life. Opening yourself up to life is part of what taking control means.

It also means—make no mistake about it—work.

What? Work? Weren't we going to get away from all that?

No, we weren't. We're getting away from diets and deprivation. But there is a difference between deprivation and work. Taking real control takes work and energy. It takes more effort and commitment, not to mention patience, than walking into the nearest diet center. But the payoff is immense.

For one thing, it works.

MAKING FOOD A PLEASURE

You want blueberry cheesecake? Go for it.

Only don't swallow, right?

Eat it, chew it, swallow it.

Just don't enjoy it? If I feel guilty enough, maybe next time I'll have brussels sprouts?

Oh, shut up and eat your cheesecake. And we mean it. If you are expecting to hear about all the things you have to do without, forget it. If you want the cheesecake, have the cheesecake and enjoy it, and then forget it and go on with your life. Chances are, if you skip the cheesecake, it will prey on your mind. You'll eat half a dozen other things to get around it. Then, eventually, you'll eat the cheesecake anyway. And you'll feel guilty and angry with yourself for giving in.

"Food is not magic," says Doris, a former Optifast client who is fifty years old. "I've heard the counselor go over this in every diet program. I'm not stupid, I know food isn't magic. Why do I like it so much?"

Maybe because it tastes good. Maybe because it's one of the simplest, sweetest pleasures life has to offer.

Every diet doctor, diet book, and diet program tells you that you should eat to live, not live to eat, that food is not pleasure, it is just fuel for the body. If you buy this, either you fell to earth from another planet or we have some swamp land . . .

There is no way you could grow up in this culture and not have some emotional connection with food. There is no way you could grow up in *any* culture and not know that eating is pleasurable. "My mother says she's bringing over some of her lasagna, it will cheer me up," says Janice, a refugee of both Weight Watchers and Nutri/System, "and, oddly enough it will. This runs against everything I am told about the right way to deal with food. I must have some real unconscious neurotic needs."

Neurotic, hell. Food is linked to every kind of human activity. It is the focus of our social lives and the center of our celebrations. But it goes much deeper than that. Food is the first pleasure a human being knows. It is the first instance of having needs met. And those needs go beyond physical hunger. Along with food comes affection, intimacy, stimulation, and comfort. This is not neurotic. This is the normal pattern of things. The fact that food is connected to so many emotional and physical states at so early an age—before words—is the reason food habits are so difficult to modify.

> When I write of hunger, I am really writing about love and the hunger for it, and warmth and the love of it and the hunger for it . . . and then the warmth and richness and fine reality of hunger satisfied . . . and it is all one.

MARY FRANCES KENNEDY FISHER

Forget blaming the mother who offered you a cookie for behaving in the grocery store, the parents who bought you candy and popcorn at the circus, the cake your grandmother made every birthday. We are talking about a connection that goes back to the day you were born. It just makes sense.

What doesn't make sense is to believe that, after a lifetime of symbolic meaning, suddenly *food will only be nourishment.* Programs and diets that sell this idea will never succeed. The only way to break the tie between food and feeling permanently is probably to have some of your brain matter removed.

We think a better way to approach this issue is to deal with reality. In reality, food *is* sometimes more than nourishment. It is comfort and nurturing. It is ritual and merrymaking. No one has ever yet tried to claim that no emotions are involved in looking at a sunset. Why pretend people can be objective about food?

So, acknowledge that you like to eat. Don't be ashamed of it. Grant that you sometimes eat for reasons other than discomfort in your abdomen and always will. Don't worry about it.

Everything else we say about food in this book will be based on this perception. Everything about feeling in control of what you eat, having a sense of increasing health, everything will be based on acknowledging and working with the place food naturally and rightfully has in your emotional and sensual life.

TRUSTING YOUR BODY

> *The body has its own way of knowing, a knowing that has little to do with logic, and much to do with truth, little to do with control, and much to do with acceptance, little to do with division and analysis, and much to do with union.*
>
> MARILYN SITWELL

There's something you may have heard a lot of lately. *Success begins with thinking your body is okay right now, no matter what you weigh.*

Don't you hate that? As if you could, right? You've spent your whole life believing, and being told by everybody around you, that you are not okay. Now, suddenly, you're supposed to turn around and think, "Hey, 175 pounds is just as beautiful as 125. And I'm just as beautiful as Jane Seymour." (Men, please substitute Mel Gibson.) *Even though all those other people haven't changed their minds.*

The people you want to date (or your spouse) would still prefer Jane Seymour. Your boss would still prefer Jane Seymour. Your mother would still prefer Jane Seymour. But you're supposed to have the strength of character to prefer yourself. Is that what we're saying?

Yes.

What?

We said, "Yes." In the first place, it's extremely unlikely that the people who know you and care about you would actually prefer you to be someone else. And even if it were true, somehow you would have to find a way to want to be you. If you buy the cultural credo that thin is better than fat, that being the way you aren't is better than being the way you are, you are seriously stuck.

Andra Medea, founder of Chimera, an organization which teaches self-defense for women, tells about a question that eventually comes up in every class she teaches. Somewhere about the middle of the class, when they are talking about methods for fighting off an attacker, one woman will hold up her hand and ask, "But what if I get tired? What if I just can't go on?" Medea replies, "You want me to tell you it's okay, to give you permission to give up, but I can't. I don't know what will happen to you if you do, but it's probably going to hurt."

We're in kind of the same position here. We'll do our best to help you find ways to accept yourself in the face of personal insecurities and cultural indoctrination, but in the end it's up to you to find the strength and the courage somewhere. Because, if you don't, it's *definitely* going to hurt.

You need to learn to trust your body again. It's part of you and who you are. Behaving as though it's some hostile stranger that you have to manipulate and deceive is no way to live. *It's also no way to lose weight.*

> *If shame could cure obesity, there wouldn't*
> *be a fat person in the world.*

SUSAN WOOLEY

Rejecting the person you are now does not help you to change. All those magazine articles saying you should put a picture of yourself looking your fat worst or your thin best on the refrigerator are just wrong. The better you feel about your body, the more likely you are to treat it well. And that's how weight gets under control.

What may be very important for you to understand is that acceptance of the person you are now, and the shape you are now, does not mean rejecting the possibility of change. It means saying, "This is one of the sizes I will be in my life. Let me see what it has to teach me and what it can give me."

Say that you are taking a vacation in Europe. You begin in London and, after visiting Barcelona, Amsterdam, Paris, and Vienna, you are going to end up in Rome. Each city is there to be explored and delighted in, giving up its secrets and its treasures . . . if you accept it as the place you are and the place you want to be. If, on the other hand, you treat it as a stopping place on the way to Rome, a place to sleep and eat and hurry on past as quickly as possible, it will give you nothing. And you may get so exhausted at having to work your way through those unpleasant places that you never get to Rome.

Now, what we're asking you to do here is very difficult. We probably won't confront you with anything more difficult in this entire book. But, in the chapters that follow, we're going to give you some help. In the meantime, give it some thought. In your life, there are different relationships with the world to be explored. Do you, at your larger weight, have certain freedoms that people who are more "marketable" in the sexual arena don't have? It's not a betrayal of your dream of a smaller body to enjoy those freedoms. You can enjoy the communication you have with other women—or other men—that is not tainted by their envy. You can explore the sense of power that size can give, instead of always hoping for the power that you think thinness might give you. You could even have fun. You could tell the cute guy in sales that he ought to burn his green sweater. He wouldn't be as mortified hearing it from someone who has a "motherly" quality as he would from the trophy blonde at reception. And it would give you a way of relating to him that she will never have. Or, if you're a man, you could use your non-threatening persona to talk to the women you work with and discover things about women that most men never have. You may even find you can keep that kind of connection to the opposite sex if and when your shape changes.

So, once again, these are the three principles of our approach: take control, accept food as a pleasure, and trust your body. Whatever helps you do these things is good, even if it's eating chocolate frosting by the spoonful. (More on that later.) Whatever stands in the way is bad, even if it's endorsed by the surgeon general, Covert Bailey, and Dr. Ruth. And that's the closest you're going to get to a "Do's and Don'ts" list in this book. (Except that we do have one really nice set of rules from Satchel Paige that we may not be able to resist.)

THE MECHANICS

Now, keep those three principles in mind while we look at the mechanics of weight control.

This is an issue that is only beginning to be understood. For a very long time, we believed that there was a simple, straightforward, and direct relationship between calorie intake/output and weight. If you took in more calories than you used up, you gained weight. If you used up more calories than you took in, you lost weight. They used to call this the bathtub theory. The calories you put into your body were the water going into the tub. The calories you used up were the calories going down the drain. If you put in more than you let out, what was left over was fat.

> *The trouble with people is not that they
> don't know but that they know so much
> that ain't so.*

JOSH BILLINGS

This is what mathematicians and scientists call an "elegant" theory. It has the virtue of utter and complete simplicity. It was diet law in the medical community for five decades.

Unfortunately it's wrong.

Wrong?

It's not as wrong as saying the earth is flat. But it's wrong enough to explain why your diet history is a mess.

What it doesn't take into consideration is your body's survival mechanisms. Covert Bailey and William Bennett both point out that people have noticed (at least, before drastic diets) that though their body weight fluctuates, they seem to have a normal center point. That is, if they overeat, they may gain weight temporarily, but when they return to a more rational diet, they go back to their usual, or *setpoint,* weight.

Similarly, a starvation diet may cause you to lose weight, but when you go back to normal eating, you quickly gain pounds and return to your original weight. The implication is that the body resists change in either direction. (No one has documented precisely how a setpoint is established early in life—though it seems to be largely hereditary—or exactly how the body knows. But it apparently works through a communication between your body's fat cells and your brain.)

**Your *setpoint* is the weight your body
thinks it should weigh.**

What tools does the body use to regulate the setpoint? Well, one of them is that old favorite, metabolism. We've probably all heard thin people brag that they have a high metabolism and fat people claim that they have a low metabolism. In the area of diet and weight control, it's a much used and abused word.

There are so many variations from one human being to another and so many factors that affect metabolism, even a medical person would be hard-pressed to say how your body handles everything you eat. But basically, your metabolism is the process that converts what you take in, food, into energy that supports all kinds of life functions, whether you're running a mile or breathing and repairing cells. And when you suddenly reduce your calorie intake, it slows down.

What happens is something like this. When you go on a diet, your body, unaware that you are kindly trying to give it a more acceptable shape, thinks you are starving and tries to help out. It says, "Okay, things are rough out there, right? You can't get enough food, right? Don't worry, I'll slow things down in here and get by on less. Everything'll be just fine. Pretty soon you'll find a better grazing ground, and I'll be working so efficiently we'll just pack that essential body fat right back on. And a little more for the next time things get rough, now that we know they can. You and me, kid, we'll get through this together."

That's perhaps a bit of an oversimplification, but you get the idea. Your body is slowing your metabolism to protect your setpoint.

> On a reduced-calorie diet, your **metabolism** slows to protect your setpoint.

In other words, trying to remain on a deprivation diet is like trying to lift a rug while you're standing on it. Your body is against you every step of the way. As William Bennett and Joel Gurin pointed out in 1982 in their classic, *The Dieter's Dilemma*, "When one's weight begins to deviate from the setpoint—as a result of dieting, say, or festive overeating—it is the brain that pulls on the reins.'' In order to defeat you, it will slow you down and make you crave food the way the old prospector crawling across the desert craves water. (A diet center puts a client into that state and then takes no responsibility when she "doesn't have the will power" to remain in the program.)

In order to lose weight, you have to deal with your setpoint. You can't get around it, you have to go through it.

> ### You must *lower your setpoint* to lose weight long term.

So how do you lower your setpoint? There is still a need for more research, but it seems that to lower your setpoint—if it can be lowered—you need to *lower your dietary fat* and increase your lean body mass. In other words, you should lighten your eating habits and *move your body as much as possible.*

Dietary fat seems to act on your body the way nuts act on squirrels. Fat comes along and your body wants to store it away for the hard times. So it slows its metabolism, making sure that as little of the fat as possible gets used for immediate energy and as much as possible gets packed on for the future. This is not true of carbohydrates. (A calorie is not a calorie is not a calorie.) If you want your metabolism to speed up, you have to stop providing your body with that tempting fat.

As for exercise, which is equally important, it seems to work like this. When you're active, your body figures you need mobility. So it burns up as much body fat as possible. Look at serious runners. The women usually have less than 15 percent body fat, and the men are sometimes as low as 5 percent body fat. All the rest is muscle/lean body mass. If you are a marathon runner, your body has the good sense to know you cannot do that twenty-six miles hauling thirty pounds of extra fat. So it will try to get rid of the fat. Just as, when you are starving, it will try to hold onto it.

How does this work? In several ways. But the most important is this: dietary fat is *burned* by muscle and *stored* by body fat. The more muscle you have, the more dietary fat you burn. The more body fat you have, the less dietary fat you burn. It is not just the number of calories the runners burn that keeps them thin. *It is the development of their lean body mass,* which then burns fat more quickly and easily.

> ### The more **muscle** you have, the more dietary fat you burn.

According to a number of researchers, there is still more to the fat-burning process. Increasing physical activity appears to increase the growth of fat-burning enzymes. These are protein molecules that grow when the body is more active. This whole process is what Covert Bailey calls, "building a better butter burner," a body primed to burn fat. (If you want to read more about this process, you might want to get a copy of *The New Fit or Fat* by Bailey. For information about the book, look in the Appendix, Resources.)

If you lower your fat intake *without drastically reducing your calorie intake,* and if you increase your activity, you will almost certainly lower your setpoint. And that means you will lose weight.

But here's where we have to remind you about the three basic principles. You can't, just can't, do these two crucial things without tackling the accumulation of emotion, symbolism, and dependency that have grown up around food and exercise in your life. If you put this book down now and put yourself on a low-fat diet, you'll soon be in as much trouble as ever. So long as you are still held captive by the diet mentality, real long-term weight loss is as far beyond your capabilities as painting the Sistine Chapel. And you free yourself from that mentality by taking control, making food a pleasure, and trusting your body.

Jane Hirschmann and Carol Munter, in their book *Over-*

coming Overeating, refer to the diet mentality as a "game" that literally becomes the shape of your life. The rules of the game are the beliefs that every committed dieter carries logged in her consciousness forever.

RULES OF THE DIET GAME

1. Fat is bad.
2. Fat people eat too much.
3. Thin is beautiful.
4. Eating requires control.
5. Criticism leads to change.

To Hirschmann and Munter's rules, we're sure you could add dozens of your own. For example:

6. Happiness is a reward for discipline.
7. French fries are a privilege, not a right.
8. Calories count.
9. No one ever got thin eating ice cream.
10. Your husband (or lover or whatever) deserves a thin body to love.
11. The best exercise is pushing yourself away from the table.
12. All vegetables are good except avocados.
13. All dairy products are bad except cottage cheese.
14. Never drink calories.

But the major, overriding, most important rule of this game is that *someone else makes up the rules.* To lose weight, you must follow a set of strict guidelines. In accordance with America's abiding faith in professional expertise, the guidelines are developed by a specialist who is wiser than you and privy to some magic you cannot possibly know. If you deviate from the plan, you are, justifiably, in for indictments, self-recriminations, and punishments.

You didn't just eat a candy bar when you were supposed to be on a diet that says no refined sugar. You made a pig of yourself. You ruined the day, maybe the week or the year. You are bad, you have blown it, you will never succeed at anything, and tomorrow you can only have juice and salad.

Right?

Let's rethink this. Perhaps candy bars have been your favorite treat since the beginning of time. So, after two weeks on The Diet, you ate one. Not six, just one. And you think this requires some sort of penance. You think there's something dreadful about that candy bar because the only success on a diet is perfect adherence. There is no room for deviation or dalliance.

To paraphrase Al Smith, no matter how thin you slice all that, it's still baloney. The Middle Ages had a word for the diet mentality. It was called asceticism. Even in those days it only worked for religious fanatics, and they mostly lived in caves.

You have to stop following other people's rules and take control of your life again. You also have to get over this hostility to your body's desires and instincts. You have to learn to trust your body again. Otherwise, self-deprivation can become a state of mind. You begin to deprive yourself not only of creamy cheeses and hot fudge sundaes, but of brightly colored clothes and dancing, of music and laughter and sex. You start feeling that you don't deserve playing in the surf or picnics in the park. You deprive yourself of life.

And you also have to stop thinking of food as a necessary evil.

There's a whole vocabulary that goes with the diet game. It's heavily larded with moral judgments. Most of the phrases in it use the words *good* and *bad*. This vocabulary adds weight and authority to the rules and makes the deprivation seem not only necessary but noble.

Well, in a first step toward taking control, toward breaking the deprivation habit and enjoying life again, here's a new glossary of terms.

cheating: A word henceforth to be used only in connection with poker, income taxes, and perhaps sexual indiscretions.

good food: The food you like to eat. Carrots are good food, so are nacho chips.

bad food: Obviously, food that is spoiled, tainted, poorly prepared, stale, or tasteless. Green cheesecake is bad food. So is food that tastes like the wrapper it came in.

good day: The day you win the Nobel Prize or an Academy Award or are named Poet Laureate, the day you hear your child's first real word, the day you find your other slipper that has been missing for two weeks and maybe, just maybe, the day you eat only a dozen cookies when a month ago you would have finished the box.

bad day: The day you discover you mistook the allergy pills for the birth control pills.

deprivation: Doing without chocolate forever, thinking you'll never see a Hostess cupcake again, eating undressed salad as your main course in your favorite French restaurant, thinking you've eaten the last Ben and Jerry's you'll ever see. Not just being forced to live on fewer than 800 calories worth of powdered milk.

ideal weight: The weight you can maintain comfortably, without eating the glue off the wallpaper, yelling at the kids for extended periods, or chasing the dog for his rawhide bone. This number cannot be found on a chart or in a computer.

perfect body: An entity which, like the unicorn, chimera, and griffin, does not exist.

scam: Any quick weight loss plan, including injections of cow placenta, the Thinking Man's Diet, the

Drinking Man's Diet, and the Doctor's Quick Weight Loss Through Sex with Celebrities the Elvis Way Diet.

To go along with your new vocabulary, we are *not* going to give you a new set of rules. In this book, there are no forbidden foods, no forbidden eating times and places, and no bad eating behaviors. And there are no other kinds of rules, restrictions, or rigid structures. Well, actually, for those of you who would feel completely lost without rules, maybe we'll throw in one or two. Like this one.

Never wear white shoes before Memorial Day or after Labor day.

What we will be giving you are some skills and techniques, ways to help you turn yourself over to yourself so that you can eat what you want when you want to, enjoy your body and be in control of your life.

Good luck. It ought to be quite an adventure.

8
Skill Number One: Reality Testing

The problem is I really don't know what I look like. If I binge the night before, I think I look fat. If I stick to my diet, I look thinner.

WORKSHOP MEMBER

IF YOU WANT to get your weight under control, you need to look, really look, at where you are now, how you got there, and what your future might be like. This is your first step in taking control.

You have large thighs, and your friend Sophia has a round belly. Carole is shaped like a pear, and Barbara has not a single straight line anywhere on her torso. George has wide, bony shoulders, and John has muscular, sloping shoulders. Our bodies are a wide variety of sizes and shapes. We are shaped like our mothers and our grandmothers—or our great-aunts. We have the Harrington hips or the Goldberg thighs. We were born to look as we look. As William Bennett, co-author of *The Dieter's Dilemma,* recently pointed out, "In the last ten years studies comparing identical with fraternal twins, adopted and biological children with their parents and twins reared apart have consistently shown that fatness is highly heritable. In a developed country, roughly two-thirds of the difference in body fat between any two people is attributable to their genes."

Not your self-indulgence. Not your lack of self-discipline. Not your inherent moral flabbiness. Your genes.

We now know that people are born with a predisposition to a certain size. We know that your body shape, like everything else, is to some degree programmed in your genes. We also know that individuals use or burn calories differently.

Unfortunately, not everything about the endocrine system is known, but there is enough evidence about metabolism to say that someone who is carrying extra fat cells does not burn calories in the same way as the naturally lean individual. Some people also have a lower proportion of "brown fat," a kind of fat that creates heat; these people also burn calories more slowly. And some people use insulin, which metabolizes sugar and other refined carbohydrates, less efficiently. These concepts help explain why some people remain fat without really trying and why some people stay thin without really trying.

This is definitely not fair. But neither is the fact that you will never sing like Beverly Sills or dance like Gregory Hines. And the same could be said about all the pluses you inherited. Is it fair that you have wonderful teeth and a knack for a good turn of phrase? Is it fair that you have perfect skin and Hilda has rampant acne? To some degree, you have to play the hand you're dealt.

However, it is unfair, discriminatory, and destructive that in our society, a woman with the Harrington hips is made to feel that she is in some significant way inferior to a woman with the Brinkley, MacPherson, or Crawford hips. Not just less attractive, but distinctly inferior. She is made to understand that society *disapproves* of the Harrington hips and thinks that, if she had sufficient character, she could "do something about them."

> The trouble with us in America isn't that the poetry of life has turned to prose, but that it has turned to advertising copy.
>
> LOUIS KRONENBERGER

This same society forgets that generations of husbands and lovers have been quite fond of the Harrington hips.

Indeed, the sexual attractiveness that we might call "personal"—that between two people in an intimate relationship—has been largely overshadowed by public judgments on a woman's physical acceptability. A man of our acquaintance said, "Any reasonably mature man is turned on by the body of the woman he loves, not the other way around." It's a simple statement, and you would probably agree that that's the way you feel about your husband or lover. But, if you're a woman, millions of dollars are spent every year to persuade you that your husband doesn't feel that way about you, that male sexuality does not work that way. And that, even if your husband *is* turned on by your body, that's not enough.

A remarkably high standard of "physical attractiveness"—read conformity to the thin aesthetic—is considered necessary in areas that are completely unrelated to the bedroom. It would be difficult to make an argument for a direct correlation between waist size and competence in a court of law. It's hard to imagine claiming that large upper arms affect the ability to audit corporate reports. And yet, presumably based on the "fat-is-weak-and-undisciplined" argument, people make those judgments every day.

IS IT UNHEALTHY TO BE OVERWEIGHT?

But, you say, isn't it unhealthy to be fat?

This is a difficult question and an enormously serious one. The medical community has been saying for so long that fat is hazardous to your health that challenging it might seem to be on a par with prescribing peach pits to treat leukemia.

But it's not. It's not even new. As far back as 1974, in his book *Fat Can Be Beautiful*, Abraham Friedman, M.D., stated, "It may surprise you to learn that people who are mildly to moderately obese and have normal blood pressure, blood sugar, and cholesterol, *have no medical cause to be concerned about their weight.*" (Emphasis Friedman's.)

Bernard Gutin, M.D., and Gail Kessler, in *The High*

Energy Factor, go further. "Obesity by itself is not a risk factor [in high blood pressure, high cholesterol level, or adult-onset diabetes]."

And in the Framingham study—one of the most respected on the long-range correlation between diet and health, particularly cardiovascular health and longevity—the findings confirmed this lack of relationship between weight and health. "Life expectancy was the *worst* for the thinnest men of Framingham," Bennett and Gurin report in *The Dieter's Dilemma.* "Above this lowest level, weight simply had little effect on the men's mortality rate. Similarly, the very lightest and the very heaviest women of Framingham had a mortality rate higher than average, but between the extremes, weight had a negligible correlation with mortality. Other projects, somewhat less ambitious than the Framingham but carefully designed and analyzed have come to the same conclusion: 'Desirable' weight is a statistical fiction."

So where do doctors get this apparently irresistible urge to tell their patients, "Drop twenty pounds or else!"?

Well, according to William Bennett, M.D., and Joel Gurin in *The Dieter's Dilemma,* the worst of it began with one actuary at the Metropolitan Life Insurance Company. He noticed one day that a lot of "fat" people died earlier than he thought they should, thereby costing his company money. He therefore went on a personal crusade to thin down America, citing a list of diseases that is still being recited today—heart disease, nephritis, diabetes, hypertension, stroke. When doctors and popular writers on weight loss go into this litany, you'll know they got it from that legendary statistician.

But what was the basis of his crusade (which garnered him a great deal of personal publicity and seems to have served as his personal vindication for some unaccepted academic work)? To begin with, all of the people in his statistical sample were owners of life insurance policies in the early part of this century. In other words, they were upper-middle- to upper-class white males. Virtually no one else had life insurance. (The Framingham study was much more representative of the American public as a whole.)

Many of these men died of the diseases in the actuary's lists. They also ate, drank, smoked, and sat on their butts in the grand tradition of the nineteenth century.

Now, in the years that have followed, research has shown each and every one of these factors—a *very* high fat diet, alcohol, smoking, and a sedentary lifestyle—to have a *causative* effect on ill health.

The same is not true for obesity.

According to the Centers for Disease Control, in 1990, the leading preventable cause of heart disease is lack of exercise. Obesity is far down the list—and a moderate amount of weight above the national average doesn't even enter in.

Some people might argue that exercise is good for you primarily because it makes you thinner. But that, apparently, is not true. Gutin and Kessler point out that exercise produces a relaxation response in the body. They make a strong argument that it is the relaxation response, *not the weight loss,* that lowers blood pressure. They also did a study comparing men of equal weight ranges on a variety of coronary risk factors. It turned out that body fat percentages, *not weight,* were good predictors of high cholesterol levels and HDL ratios and of coronary heart disease.

That is to say, your heart doesn't benefit from weight loss; it benefits from exercise that relaxes you and makes you fitter.

It is, perhaps, understandable that doctors might mistake a symptom—obesity—for the disease itself—lack of fitness—but it leads to disastrous results, for one very simple reason. Becoming more fit may decrease your risk of illness, but dieting to lose weight will almost certainly *increase* it.

That's right, increase it. Dieting destroys muscle cells, including muscle cells in the heart. And that weakens your heart.

In an article entitled ''Change in Body Weight and Longevity'' in the *Journal of the American Medical Association* in the fall of 1992, I. Lee and R. S. Paffenberger demonstrated that, according to the JAMA abstract, ''weight loss *increases* cardiovascular mortality, even in overweight subjects. Weight fluctuation increased mortality by over 50 percent, which overshadows the 18 percent rise in mortality associated with the top quintile of obesity."

In other words, even the most obese people have much less risk of dying of a heart attack than people who diet.

In fact, Reubin Andres, M.D., of the National Institute of Aging, states, "Limited weight gain during the adult years is associated with favorable survival experiences" and cites ten studies on the long-term effects of change in weight to prove his point that "mortality is lowest in the segment of the population that gained some weight during the adult years." (Andres concedes that weight loss due to illness and cigarette smoking may affect these statistics.)

So why does your doctor tell you to lose weight? Well, according to C. Wayne Callaway, M.D., adviser on the federal government's "1990 Dietary Guidelines for Americans," it's because he or she is a victim of antifat prejudice. "Doctors who feel deep down that women are supposed to be thin will have a hard time with the new notion that some extra weight isn't bad," says Callaway.

John Mead, M.D., director of the Adolescent and Young Adult Eating Disorder Program at Rush-Presbyterian St. Luke's Medical Center in Chicago, concurs. "Antifatism is alive and well in the health care profession," he says, after testing hundreds of health care workers for prejudice.

Another reason is ignorance. Most internists, gynecologists, and general practitioners simply do not know enough about bariatrics to understand that there is virtually no such thing as permanent weight loss from dieting. When they say, "Lose a little weight. What could it hurt?" they really don't know.

We're not saying that you should simply ignore what your doctor has to say, or even that you should dismiss arbitrarily anyone who brings up in print the question of weight loss for health. But we are suggesting that you should exercise caution and judgment. There is often an almost hysterical tone in the warnings against obesity. So look for these signs of knee-jerk weight loss advice:

- a list of diseases supposedly caused by obesity, without research to establish the connections

- use of the words *obese* and *overweight* interchangeably and without clear definition

- sweeping statements about an epidemic of obesity in the United States, again without a clear definition of what that condition is

- outdated advice about diet, rather than fitness and setpoint

- recommending weight loss for people with a somewhat above-average amount of fat and defending that recommendation by referring to statistics about the morbidly obese, those whose body fat percentage is 50 to 70 percent

This last point is very important. Even if dieting is not the answer to their problem, there *are* people who carry more weight than is good for them. But you can't tell by weighing them. Their danger is a factor of the *percentage of fat* in their bodies, not their weight. And that percentage has to be considerably higher than that of the average diet center customer.

Most of you are simply not obese.

An article in the June 1993 issue of *Consumer Reports* reviews the major diet programs and says, "The women in those programs averaged 167 pounds when they started and a body mass index of 28. . . . A body mass index of 25 or less is considered desirable, while most people with a body mass index of over 30 are considered seriously overweight."

We would argue that, even here, the term "seriously overweight" is misused. You will notice that, in this book, we try not to use the word *overweight*. This is not simply because it implies a value judgment (overweight implies weighing more than you *should*). Also, it is a nebulous, imprecise, and virtually meaningless word. We try to say, instead, exactly what we mean in any given context; for example, "above the national average" or "above the weight you would like to be." As for obesity, we use it to mean a percentage of body fat near or above fifty.

To make this more concrete and put the whole question

of weight and health into perspective, let's look at an example. Janet is forty-five years old. She is five feet, six inches tall and weighs 180 pounds. Her blood pressure and blood sugar are normal, her cholesterol below normal. The average doctor would probably tell her she should lose some weight. Should she?

Well, even the most diehard members of the medical establishment seldom claim that anyone is running a health risk who weighs less than 20 percent more than his or her "desirable" weight. These people are often unclear about what that desirable weight is supposed to be, but we'll use the latest weight tables issued by the federal government. Janet's weight, according to these charts, is within the desirable range at 167. Twenty percent above that would be 200 pounds.

Janet's fine. And if she believes her doctor and starts dieting, she could ruin her health.

THE PROBLEM WITH FAT IS NOT HEALTH

But if fat is not a health problem for most of us, what kind of problem is it? Unfortunately, it is a personal, professional, social, sexual, and emotional problem. And its causes lie not just in our bodies, but in the body politic. Affluent America itself has an eating disorder.

The tragedy of this is not just that we have women who cannot believe their lovers desire them. It is not just that we have competent professionals who are denied promotions. The tragedy is that we have people—both men and women—who should be concentrating their energies on loving, rearing children, writing important books, designing beautiful buildings, growing splendid gardens, and discovering the cure for another form of cancer who are instead trying to get rid of the Harrington hips.

Unless we are willing to concede parallels to the final years of the Roman Empire and throw in the towel, we need to do something about a society in which tens of thousands of young men—thirteen and up—were recently having silicone implants in their pectorals to make them look more like Arnold Schwarzenegger, where, according to the National Association of Anorexia Nervosa and Associated Disorders, about 8 million people suffer from anorexia and other eating disorders, where one in every five college women is the victim of an eating disorder, where a highly successful attorney who weighs about twenty pounds more than the average woman can say to her diet counselor, "The most important thing in my life is how my body looks."

In the meantime, however . . .

In the meantime, you have to get through your life. You can't wait until society comes around to a healthier way of looking at people and their images. Reality testing will help you see *whether* you need to alter your body size, *why* you may think you need to change, and *what forces* you will be dealing with emotionally, physically, and socially in trying to come to grips with this issue.

YOUR PHYSIOLOGICAL LEGACY

In the next few pages, you'll find two questionnaires that are designed to help you analyze the complex factors that make up your relationship with your body and with food.

First you need to try to decide what shape and size is physiologically realistic for you, as opposed to what is culturally imposed. This involves looking at your family, at the weight you were before you started dieting, and at other factors that might give you a clue as to the size that would be most comfortable for you. The weight your body wants to be and tries very hard to be—your setpoint—is easier to change than your height or glove size, but not much. (In other words, Jane Fonda will probably always be thinner than you are.)

You can't find your setpoint by looking at a chart. And the diet centers can't find it by plugging numbers into a computer, much as they try to make you think they can. You have to consider many complex factors.

You also need to look at your own diet history and your present lifestyle to see what is personally possible. If you have been dieting for only a few years, have a large disposable income with which to hire a personal trainer, and have time to spend several hours a day working out, you are going to be able to make a greater change in your setpoint than a lifelong dieter with a job, three children, and no room in the family budget for fooling around. (In other words, Jane Fonda will probably always be thinner than you are.)

You probably need to see what approximation to "perfection" you can try to accept. For this one, you'll have to give some thought to what you have at stake emotionally. What does a thin body represent to you? What makes you think it's so important? Or, to put it another way, *who* makes you think it's so important? How much of your desire for a "better" body comes from inside you? Is there any way to change your expectations rather than your weight? (In other words, is there any way you could not really *care* if Jane Fonda is thinner than you are?)

If you don't think you can live with the size you are, you have to decide how big a commitment you are willing to—and can—make to change. If your size is inherited, and not just the result of too much dieting, the commitment may have to be a big one. One currently popular proponent of strenuous exercise, Susan Powter, presents herself as a model for weight loss. She went from over 200 pounds to a svelte, muscular body. But she has had to devote her entire life—including her occupation—to the effort. As she puts it, she "sweats for a living." Can you quit your job as a clerk and become an aerobics teacher? Will you? For some of you, the answer may be yes. For the others, her solution will just not work, not if you were born to be large.

Reality testing requires you to question everything you have taken for granted, everything you've been conditioned to believe about food, about weight, and about yourself.

It is not easy to erase old tapes. Aunt Helen's voice is still echoing in your mind, saying, "You would be beautiful, if you would only lose twenty pounds." The family doctor's face is before you grimacing each time he records your weight, while he points out, "if you don't do something now, you'll be forty pounds overweight in a couple of years.'' But taking control of your life means acknowledging these influences and then realizing that Aunt Helen was a horse's patoot and the family doctor knew as much about the connection between health and weight as he knew about sex education.

Questionnaire #1
Weight and Physical History

Your Family

1. How many members of your family are above average in weight and who are they?

2. Is any other member not large but always on a restricted diet? Who?

3. What is the general size and shape of the women (or men) in your family—tall, broad, square, round, apple, pear? This includes grandmothers, great-grandmothers, aunts, and so forth.

4. How did your grandmother look at thirty, forty, or fifty? How did your mother look at your age?

Yourself

5. At what age did you begin to feel that you were ''overweight''?

6. Why did you think you were ''overweight''? (Did your family, friends, or doctor make you feel self-conscious? Did you compare yourself to images in the media?)

Your First Diet

7. What did you weigh the first time you dieted?

8. How did you lose weight? Did you make up your own diet, go on a diet program, take pills, go to a doctor, cut back portions, cut out certain foods or food groups?

9. How much did you lose?

10. How long was it before you started gaining the weight back?

11. What did your weight go up to after the diet?

Your Diet History

12. How many diets have you been on since the first one?

13. What is the most weight you have lost and gained?

14. What is the lowest weight you have ever maintained comfortably for a long period?

15. Are you aware of changes in your eating habits since you went on the first diet? List any.

16. How much do you know about your eating habits? Have you ever kept a journal?

17. How does your present weight compare with your weight when you first dieted?

Your Body Type

18. At what weight do you presently feel physically, not emotionally, comfortable? (That means you can walk briskly without huffing and puffing or climb a flight of stairs with ease.)

19. Is most of your excess weight carried in one area of your body? Where?

20. Are you broad in either the shoulders or the hips? What size are your hands, wrists, and feet?

What Do Your Answers Mean?

The purpose of this inventory is to figure out your predisposition to be a particular size or weight. All right, look at the first six questions. What picture do you now have of your family? Are they mostly tall, slender types? Do they tend to gain weight in their forties? Do most of the women have large busts or large hips? What's the silhouette you're starting to see? This is important. If you've been thinking that the only difference between your round, matronly grandmother and Marlene Dietrich is that Dietrich didn't "let herself go," you've probably been doing your grandmother an injustice.

We're not saying that you have to be exactly the same shape as everybody else in your family. However, if you come from a long line of zaftig women, you're going to have to work very hard to vary from that tradition. And you won't vary very much. You should be asking yourself at this point exactly why you want to change. Where did you get the idea that the way you look is not good enough?

YOUR DIET HISTORY

Now consider the next group of questions, concerning your diet history. The answer to the first one is, for a remarkable number of women, their ideal setpoint or something very close to it. The exception is the woman who went on her first diet after a period of eating *above her setpoint*. For example, if you weighed somewhere near 130 through high school and, during your first year in college, went up to 140, you probably spent those first free months away from home indulging in pizza four times a week and lots of vending machine junk food. If you had just gone back to eating more sensibly and been patient, the ten pounds would have disappeared. (Of course, if you continued that pattern for an extended period, your body would manufacture new fat cells and your setpoint would go up, but that wouldn't happen in six or eight months.) In that case, your original setpoint was the 130 you weighed at seventeen rather than the 140 you weighed at nineteen.

You should also be looking at how extreme your first diet was. Did you starve yourself and lose twenty-five pounds in two months? If so, was your regaining the weight just as extreme? If you went more slowly, did the weight come back more slowly? This gives you a picture of your body before you altered its setpoint and its fat percentage by dieting.

Now, look at your diet history. The less extreme your dieting has been, the better chance you have that you will be able to overcome the bad effects on your body. The more extreme it has been, the more difficult a task you are facing. With each diet, you have almost certainly altered the proportion of fat to lean body mass. And, as you became "overfat," your body took on more fat more easily. And your setpoint rose.

Finally, look at your body type. Forget about all those measurements the magazines used to ask you to take. You know, if your wrists are between five and six inches, you have a small frame, that sort of thing. Just use your common sense. If you're a broad-shouldered woman with feet that are size nine, you're probably not going to weigh the same as a narrow-shouldered woman who wears a size five.

Let's take an example. You are five six and weigh 150 pounds. Your mother and maternal grandmother are both roundish women and your father sports a pretty good set of love handles. When you went on your first diet, you weighed 130. You dieted down to 120 in a month and then went back up to 135 within four months. You've been on half a dozen diets in the four or five years since then. Each time, you've ended up a few pounds heavier. You're not particularly broad-shouldered, but you've always been a little wide in the hips. Your setpoint right now may be close to your present weight of 150. There is still the chance that you might be able to get your setpoint down to near where you started out, at 130, altering the percentage of your body fat by increasing your movement and lowering the amount of fat in your diet. Going below that, however, would mean a level of exercise you may not be willing to commit to.

Questionnaire #2
Family Behavior About Food

1. What memories do you have about food and family? Write a couple of paragraphs about the importance of food in your home, atmosphere at mealtimes, celebrations and food, and availability of food.

2. Did food seem an important matter to other family members?

3. Was food offered as a reward for good behavior?
4. Were there lots of rules or prohibitions related to food or mealtimes in your house? Write down anything you remember. For example, did you get a choice at meals? Were you allowed snacks, candy, soda? Did you have to finish everything on your plate?
5. Were family members health-conscious about food?
6. Were meals prepared for you, or did you have to take care of yourself?
7. How would you rate your family's eating habits and attitude toward food? Healthy? Obsessive? Indifferent?
8. Did you observe ways, other than eating, of dealing with stress and tension in your family? Did people in your family get mad, go for a walk, go to the driving range to hit a bucket of balls, have a drink?
9. How much did your family identify as positive attributes other than physical appearance? What skills, talents, or interests were valued?
10. Was physical activity an important part of family events? Did you often take a walk or go biking or skiing together rather than sitting in front of the television?

What Do Your Answers Mean?
The answers to these questions are very personal and will be different for each one of you, but they should give you some idea of how important a role food played in your family's social interaction, to what degree food was a part of your family glue.

Perhaps mealtimes were when everyone met and talked about what was happening in their lives. Or perhaps most meals were lonely events, when your parents were at work. Perhaps they were times of conflict, when the tensions of family life rose to the surface and power games were played over the roast. These things affect how you feel about food.

Home is the place where eating habits and attitudes begin to form. Those habits are probably still with you, standing between you and the kind of freedom you want and need, no matter how old you are. You may still feel it is sinful to waste food. You may have an absolute compulsion to eat "what is good for you" in order to earn the reward of dessert. If you're hungry at four, you may still resist snacking, even though that is the only way to keep yourself from falling on your dinner like a timber wolf.

These are things you need to make yourself aware of. Once you do, you can start to operate with more freedom. You need to be able to break habits, break rules, and break out of the restrictions that have locked you in for so long.

It may also help to understand why controlling your weight is so important to you.

SUGGESTIONS

1. If your doctor is not sensitive to and aware of newer findings about weight, consider finding one who is. If you want to stick with the one you have, give him or her a copy of this book. (This will have the added advantage of increasing our royalties.)

2. Start looking everywhere to discover what real people look like. Look at the grocery store, the laundry, and the playground. Don't do this competitively, asking yourself if you look better than other people or if they look better than you. Do it with openness and affection for all the ways human beings can look.

3. If you're a woman, choose a woman of your acquaintance whom you and others consider attractive and who weighs about as much as you do. Say her name is Janis. Then, every time you think, "The reason that guy [or my lover or my husband] is not paying attention to me is that I'm fat," or "The reason I didn't get that promotion is that I'm fat," put Janis in your place. If you decide the person

would pay attention to Janis, that Janis would get the promotion, then it's not your weight that's standing in your way. Look at other possibilities. If you're a man, you can do the same thing, focusing on your own particular areas of concern.

9
Skill Number Two:
Self-Acceptance

I guess I am just never going to be satisfied with my body. I look at the fashion magazines, forget it. No diet is going to make me look that way. Why do I keep trying?

DIET CENTER CLIENT

ONCE UPON A TIME, you and your body got along pretty well. It was what you got around in. You considered it an okay instrument for getting up a tree and, when you got a new pair of tennis shoes, you knew it was as fast as the wind. You believed what your body said to you. When it was hungry, you ate. When it was not, most of the time, you didn't. When it was tired, you slept, unless your parents let you stay up to watch a late TV show. The only time you thought about changing your body was when it wouldn't do something you wanted it to do. Like fly.

And then, if you were a girl, something happened. You got a little older. People around you started paying more attention to what your body looked like than what it did. It was no longer such a big deal that you could get to the top of the elm tree faster than anybody else. Now it was a big deal that you didn't have breasts yet—or that you did. Now some people said you were too skinny or too fat, and it had nothing to do with whether you could squeeze through the window if somebody forgot the keys to the front door.

Gradually, there was a complete reevaluation of you and your peers. Once there was Paula-who's-good-at-tetherball and Janna-who's-really-nice and Kim-who-can-put-her-foot-behind-her-neck and Jody-who-can-really-draw and Nettie-whose-Dad-is-the-principal. Now there was a mass of girls who were distinguished from each other in only one way. If you were conventionally pretty, you were at the top of the pecking order. If you weren't, you were at the bottom. Period.

It was confusing for everybody. The pretty girls didn't know how this sudden prestige got dropped in their laps, but they sure weren't going to let it go. They put on makeup and spent hours on their hair and begged their parents for the right clothes. The plain girls didn't know why they were suddenly in no man's land, but they sure weren't going to stay there. *They* put on makeup and spent hours on their hair and begged their parents for the right clothes.

And what about the fat girls?

Well, they were at the very bottom of the heap and what's more, it was their own fault. You might not be able to change the shape of your nose—unless your folks had lots of money and were, like, really nice—but you could always lose weight. The magazines said so. Your parents said so. Even your doctor said so. And as for the kids at school . . .

In our culture, a woman's alienation from her body usually begins right around puberty or a little before. Up to that time, the body passes muster pretty well because it's being judged on how well it does what you want it to do. But, because of the peculiar nature of modern American sexuality, the bodies of adult women are judged by a different standard. Their primary function is to serve as erotic inspirations to men, *visual* erotic inspirations. In other words, we're being valued for our sexuality and, not only that, our bodies are not even judged by how well they make love. They're judged by whether, when a man looks at them, *he wants* to make love to them.

Women who measure up to this standard are, according to conventional wisdom, most valuable on the marriage market. And nowadays, by a kind of weirdly American association of ideas, they're also most valuable on the job market.

The result of all this is that women in our culture develop a strange relationship with their own bodies, often marked by a fair amount of fear and hostility. We are not at home in our bodies. Far more than men, we see our bodies as less attractive than others see them. We are more dissatisfied than men with the size and shape of our bodies. It is true that, recently, that gap between men and women has been narrowed, but in the wrong way. Today, more and more, men are developing a self-consciousness about their bodies that can result in alienation.

> *The tragedy of our time is that we are so*
> *eye centered, so appearance besotted.*
>
> JESSAMYN WEST

These negative feelings are usually suppressed, but this armed peace can break out into open warfare if you get started dieting. And, unfortunately, as we pointed out earlier, there are a lot of people with a stake in your dissatisfaction with your body. A hell of a lot of money is being made by companies who sell ways for you to "fix" the way you look. We're not talking here just about diet centers. The whole beauty industry is out there offering images that make you feel inadequate in order to sell you products you don't need.

THE TYRANNY OF PERFECT BEAUTY

Listen to Beverly Johnson, one of the supermodels who has recently spoken out about eating disorders in the profession. She's discussing her thirteen-year-old daughter, who is starting to model, with a *People* magazine interviewer.

"One of these days my daughter will be in *Vogue* magazine, she will weigh 105 lbs. and pose in a dress that a 35-year-old woman will then want to buy. That's really unfair. It does a lot of damage to women's self-esteem because it makes them try to reach a goal that they will never reach."

And why should they? Why should a grown woman want to have the body of a thirteen-year-old? To take it a step further, why should there exist a profession in which thirteen-year-olds are made up to look like women and women have to starve themselves and submit to surgery in order to present an image of "perfection" that will make other women feel bad? In the same article, another top model, Carol Alt, said, "When we started in the business, you couldn't fit into the clothes if you had any breasts at all. They would bind us up. Now all the girls are getting implants." (Or were, until implants were banned. Now flat—or waiflike—is back.)

Both Johnson and Alt revealed serious eating disorders that they developed *in order to* represent the American ideal of beauty.

And where did this ideal come from anyway?

In the 1890s, it was Lillian Russell. In the teens, it was Theda Bara. In the twenties, it was flappers like Clara Bow, Louise Brooks, and Colleen Moore. In the thirties, it was Harlow, Garbo, Crawford, and Davis. The forties brought Betty Grable and Ingrid Bergman, and Katharine Hepburn came into her own. Queens of the fifties were Lana Turner, Ava Gardner, Jane Russell, Marilyn Monroe, and—odd woman out—Audrey Hepburn. At the beginning of the sixties, our ideals of beauty were Sophia Loren, Elizabeth Taylor, Grace Kelly, and Kim Novak. These were women with many styles of beauty and bodies of many sizes and shapes.

And then, sometime in the late sixties and early seventies, things began to change. All the movie stars moved over as a stick-thin Londoner named Twiggy batted her three pairs of false eyelashes and introduced the Age of the Models.

Suddenly, our idea of beauty was being derived, not from the wide variety of shapes and sizes that actresses and singers and tap dancers come in, but from advertising. Models. Women whose primary function is to make ready-made clothes look good.

Thin women.

> *All God's children are not beautiful. Most of God's children are, in fact, barely presentable.*
>
> FRAN LEBOWITZ

We've been stuck with them ever since. Ask someone for an example of a beautiful, desirable woman. Ten to one, the answer won't be Meryl Streep but Christie Brinkley, Elle MacPherson, Kim Alexis, or whoever is on the cover of this year's *Sports Illustrated* swimsuit issue. Our image of beauty is no longer a real, though thoroughly glamorized, woman moving across a stage or screen for a couple of hours, sitting, walking, bending, and falling occasionally into an awkward position that shows a little fold at the waist. It is a model who spends every waking moment keeping herself thin and who is captured for an instant and presented on paper after thirty-five inferior images have been thrown away in the darkroom.

Even Julia Roberts isn't considered good enough for that kind of image. They hired a body double to do her famous *Pretty Woman* poster. They needed perfection.

So now it's become part of our cultural belief that perfection is desirable and attainable and that perfect means thin. Advertising shows us this. Television reflects it. And the diet industry encourages it.

We don't want to oversimplify and suggest that trying to fit a fashionable stereotype started in 1965. There were, indeed, Victorian women who had ribs removed to attain an hourglass figure. And everybody knows how many diet pills Judy Garland took. Still, the pressure to get thin and stay thin is greater than it has ever been in history. Resisting the pressure to feel that you don't measure up is very difficult. It requires more than just the determination not to pay attention.

Questionnaire #3
Appearance and Self-Worth

1. Who are three women you consider really beautiful?
2. How would you describe yourself?
3. Do you think you're graceful?
4. Do you feel that you express your personality in the way you carry yourself?
5. What's the prettiest part of your body?
6. What are some of the things you do to play up your best features?
7. Do you think you would look better in the clothing of a different period in history?
8. When was the last time you felt proud of a physical accomplishment? What was it?

What Do Your Answers Mean?

Suppose you answered the first question with these three names: Elizabeth Taylor, Ava Gardner, and Sophia Loren. If you then said, in answer to the second question, that you have dark hair, strong features, and a rounded figure, your self-image is in pretty good shape. If, on the other hand, you gave the same answer to the first question and answered the second by saying that you are blond, blue-eyed, and have a sort of aristocratic charm, there's too big a gap between what you see in yourself and what you admire in other women. That indicates that you may be having trouble accepting yourself.

The next questions ask you to think about your body in terms other than weight or the usual issues of appearance. Think, too, about the way you move. Grace and confidence can be enormously attractive, can be more important to your attractiveness than losing two inches off your hips.

Your personality, as it is expressed in your carriage, your smile, and your body language, can be impressive, sexy, charming, you name it.

There was a time when a woman could be greatly admired for having soft, round shoulders. Today, while they may not be exhibited to advantage in the clothes you wear to the office, soft, round shoulders are still lovely and sexy and quite sufficient to inspire amorous thoughts. So, if you have them, appreciate them, instead of ignoring them while you focus angrily on a thick waist. And show them off. Don't focus on the negative, hiding your upper arms. If you dress only to hide what you think is "bad," the best you'll ever look is "not bad."

Find out how to dress your body at all of its sizes. If you're dressing the body you have as though it were the body you hope to have someday, you're wearing somebody else's clothes. On the other hand, if you're choosing clothes that you believe make you look as thin and as inconspicuous as possible, you're just not having any fun.

"I really got in the habit of wearing black and baggy," says Tina, an artist in her late forties who has had trouble adjusting to middle-aged weight gain. "Then one night I sort of felt daring, so I got out a couple of gauzy Indian cotton skirts I used to wear—they have drawstring waists, you know—and layered them with a bright, low-cut shirt and a *lot* of jewelry. I asked Tim how I looked. He said, 'Great!' I mean, he was really enthusiastic. Then I asked him didn't he think I looked fat. And he said, 'That's not what you asked me. The outfit doesn't make you look thin. It makes you look good.' "

BEYOND PHYSICAL BEAUTY

And don't just do better by your outsides. Do better by your whole self.

Don't save up life experiences until you're thin. You can go on a vacation to a working ranch now *and* when you have a smaller body. You'll be able to do some things better now and some things better later. Find out what both experiences have to offer. You can visit the art museum now as a dedicated art lover and later as a someone actively looking for an attractive fellow art lover.

> *Flops are a part of life's menu and I've never been a girl to miss out on any of the courses.*

> ROSALIND RUSSELL

There's a book that may help you in this process of exploring and enjoying the shape you have now. When Susie Orbach first published *Fat Is a Feminist Issue* in the late seventies, it was revolutionary. Orbach presented the shocking theory that women may *choose* fat as a response to an oppressive world. The book included a lot of exercises designed to help you discover the tasks your size might be accomplishing for you. You might, for example, feel less frail and physically at risk when you are larger. You might feel safer from unwanted attention. This book is a good conversation starter in support groups.

It's hard to see the totality of body and self. The desire for beauty is not skin-deep in most American women. Appearance is the *major* area in which we are encouraged to excel. Unfortunately, trying to excel in this area often takes away energy that you need for other things in life. On the other hand, focusing on some other area in which you can accomplish and achieve often takes the pressure off this one. There are many other aspects of self that can bring enormous pleasure into your life, if you can get beyond your appearance. Let's face it, Jane Austen didn't have buns of steel. Neither did Eleanor Roosevelt, Jane Addams, Ida B. Wells, Golda Meir, Dorothy Parker, Gertrude Stein, Sojourner Truth, Betty Ford, Mary Cassatt . . .

A 1986 Glamour *survey of thirty-three thousand women revealed that the majority chose losing ten to fifteen pounds above success in work or in love as their most desired goal.*

Think about someone you know, or have known, and respect. Ask yourself how much that person's appearance mattered to you. Would you have valued your inspiring tenth-grade English teacher more if she had weighed less? Do you have an appearance double standard? Do you judge everybody else in the world by one standard and yourself by another? What would happen in your life if you gave up the desire to be perfect and allowed your personality to have its own way?

Trying to be perfect is incredibly limiting. It leaves no room for eccentricity, creativity, rebellion, or nonconformity. Perfection is completely conventional and ultimately boring. And it's not necessary.

The world is a difficult and scary place. Some of us attempt to protect ourselves from its dangers by trying to live inside an armor of perfection, of accomplishment and achievement in every area of life. We work very hard at trying to keep all of these areas under control. When one of them starts to slip away from us, it can assume a frightening importance in our lives.

Questionnaire #4
Image and Excellence

1. In your family, how much emphasis was put on excelling?

2. Were you and your siblings expected to excel in either athletics or academics?

3. As a young person, did you feel that excellence in one area would be considered sufficient?

4. If you went to college, at what age did you start thinking about what college you would go to?

5. Did your mother pay a great deal of attention to her appearance?

6. Were your father's expressions of affection to your mother and to you often tied to comments about appearance?

7. Are you surprised when you see attractive or suc-

cessful people with partners whom you do not consider attractive?

8. Are you very conscious of clothing and the way it
affects the image you present to the world?

9. How many of the moments in your life that you
remember as intensely embarrassing have been connected to the way you looked or were dressed?

10. Do you feel more powerful when you are larger or
when you believe you look attractive?

What Do Your Answers Mean?
Your answers to this questionnaire may help you explore
the degree to which you connect your physical image with
emotional needs, especially the need to excel. In a family
in which achievement is important, appearance often becomes a focus for girls because it is an area in which
women are expected to excel. As unrelated as college
plans and appearance seem to be, the fact is that eating
disorders are unusually common among white, middle- to
upper-middle-class young women in college or on their
way. The desire to excel is simply being expressed in two
different ways.

Well, depending on your body to support your self-
esteem is risky business for anyone, even Arnold Schwarzenegger. In order to take control of your life, you may very
well have to change the way you view yourself and shift
the emphasis away from your shape.

> *There's a rule, I think. You get what you
> want in life, but not your second choice,
> too.*
>
> ALISON LURIE

To some degree, that may be a matter of establishing
priorities. You have probably believed in the past, con-
sciously or unconsciously, that you could, and should, be
successful at everything in your life. *That is not true.* It
is not true for anyone in the world. Everyone has to make

choices. And people who refuse to make choices, who try to have it all, frequently fail to accomplish much in any area or, if they do, fail to enjoy it. You may have to choose between living a happy and fulfilling life and being thin.

Ask yourself, could you put the emphasis now on other aspects of your life, and lose weight, if it's possible, later? That's what Edie decided to do.

Edie is an artist in her thirties. Her husband is a few years older, also an artist, and well established in his field. Both have struggled with weight problems all their lives. In recent years, Edie's husband seemed to be getting his weight under control, but Edie was still unhappy with hers. She is an extremely attractive and appealing woman who carries "extra" weight on her hips. She is also the daughter of a woman who puts great emphasis on appearance, especially on being slender.

In her early thirties, Edie began to experience the most severe form of premenstrual syndrome. It lasts from ovulation to menses—two weeks out of every month—and includes depression, irritability, anxiety, and food cravings. Within a couple of years, Edie's weight had gone up significantly.

While participating in a diet workshop, Edie looked carefully at her life. She reviewed her priorities and realized that the two at the very top of her list had nothing to do with her weight. She wanted to enjoy her life with her husband and she wanted to develop her career in the arts. Taking on the overwhelming task of trying to lose weight in the face of her PMS could only erode her ability to focus on those priorities.

Edie's plan of action was simple. She started walking regularly to keep herself healthy. (It has the added advantage of taking the edge off of her PMS.) She and her husband also started watching their fat intake, but Edie didn't focus on food. She focused on developing artistic projects and spending more time with Weldon. Somewhere down the line, when the PMS is over or controlled by new discoveries in medical science, Edie may consider putting more energy into weight control.

And then again, she may not. With a lot of support from her husband and friends, Edie is in the process of accepting herself as she is, and that includes large hips.

In one sense, it seems obvious that Edie would rather be a successful artist and a happily married woman than a size eight. But, in this society, the decision she made is a difficult one. Edie was helped by a good support group and a husband who, because of his own experience as an "overweight" child and adolescent, had some insight into her anxieties.

The next questions on the questionnaire deal with appearance and love. Unfortunately, for many women, there seems to be an emotional connection between excellence and lovability. We believe that we will be loved only if we are excellent, perhaps perfect. The fact that the world is littered with people who are in love with thoroughly imperfect other people doesn't penetrate our noggins. Somebody probably loved Attila the Hun.

Love that is real grows out of human qualities and feelings that have nothing to do with accomplishment or physical perfection. Everybody knows that, but some of us don't believe it. "I went back and read a bunch of love letters my husband wrote me in the first couple of years after we met," says Barb, an attractive woman who has been married for fifteen years. "There'd been so much, I guess you'd call it passion. And he did say in the letters I was sexy. But about ten times more than that he talked about warmth, tenderness, understanding, having fun together, things like that. I was really surprised."

The last few questions have to do with a kind of fear that many of us have, a fear of being vulnerable to the criticism, scorn, or laughter of others. When that fear becomes exaggerated, it can be crippling. We may be able to take any other kind of risk in life. We can stand up to dislike, anger, or moral condemnation. We can climb mountains, invest our life savings in a cookie business, or march to end wars. What we can't do is risk having anyone pity us or snicker behind our backs.

Getting over it is one of the first steps to taking real control of your life.

Since the way other people perceive you is important to you, try doing a reality check. Sit down and talk with significant people in your life, such as your spouse, lover, parents, and best friend. Tell them that you do not expect to change significantly from the shape you are now, and tell them what you intend to focus on instead. If they have concerns about your health, address them by explaining what you plan to do in that area.

Now. Did anyone freak out?

The chances are very good that they didn't, that your weight is a much bigger deal to you than to any of them. That should help to take some of the pressure off. Also, if they're warned, your friends and family may be able to help you, instead of asking how much weight you've lost on your new diet.

If you got a negative response, you're in a different situation. Perhaps more than a little of the pressure you feel to meet a certain standard of appearance is coming from outside you. That complicates matters. You're going to have to declare your emotional independence in this area, and you're probably going to need some support to do it. It will help to find other people who put less emphasis on meeting a certain narrow standard of attractiveness.

We strongly suggest that you investigate the idea of a support group. If the people in your daily life are culture-bound and cannot see beyond the thinness standard, your confidence is going to be continually eroded. To counteract that, you need a group of people whom you see regularly and who share your sense that self-worth is based on more important things than numbers on a scale.

You can also help your family and friends deal with your change in perspective by changing the way you talk about yourself. You may be using self-denigrating humor to try to minimize your embarrassment, but that kind of comment gives the people around you the cue to focus on your weight. One woman we know who has overcome this pattern said, "Once I decided this was going to be my size, I stopped talking about it. I don't bring it up with friends and I don't make jokes or comments." And neither does anyone else.

SUGGESTIONS

1. Put together a support group. Sharing your concerns and working with others within the safety of this type of group can be very freeing. And creating a small community that supports values different from those of the mainstream can be critical to growth, as anyone who belonged to a "rap group" in the early years of the women's movement will attest. You need to be around other people who are rejecting images in favor of something more real and more substantial.

2. Take control of your environment by clearing your closet of things that look good on you only when you are at your lowest weight. For the foreseeable future, those tight waistbands and unzippable zippers are going to be shame-producing, and you don't need that. Shame leads to diets, not confidence and control.

3. Get rid of all your fashion magazines and don't buy any more. They are making money off your insecurities. Besides, you don't need to spend your time looking at pictures of "ideal" bodies. If you like to read women's magazines—and still want makeup tips—buy magazines like *Self, Healthy Woman,* and *Shape* that are less exploitative and focus more on staying fit than staying thin.

4. Get a subscription to *Big Beautiful Woman.* For many of us, flipping through its pages is like being at home in the world for the first time in a long time.

5. Throw a costume party. Wear a costume from some period in history when your figure type was in style, something that makes the absolute most of your best features.

6. Put away any pictures of how "wonderful you would look if you lost weight." It's counterproductive to liking yourself in the present. Do not, *under any circumstances,* put pictures of thin women on

your refrigerator. If you want to put up pictures for inspiration, choose women who are about the size you are now and who are dressed with flair and style and look great.

7. Shop where the clothes are not styled and sized for skinny teenagers.

8. Get rid of your scale.

10
Skill Number Three: Unrestricting Your Eating

༁═

*I think I'd feel less guilt about robbing a
bank than eating a french fry.*

DIET PROGRAM CLIENT

DO YOU REMEMBER a faraway time when you ate fried
chicken, mashed potatoes with gravy, corn on the cob drip-
ping with butter and salt, and finished off with apple pie
à la mode?

Were you fatter then than you are now?

Through years of dieting, you've managed to rob yourself of a lot of great-tasting food. And you haven't got
much worth talking about in return. So take it back. Take
back some of those wonderful foods of yesteryear.

You can begin by not bad-mouthing them. Food is not
capable of theological error. So don't talk about sinful ice
cream or evil french fries. Stop seeing moral superiority
in raw vegetables. Salad does not bring you nearer to
sainthood than grilled cheese sandwiches. Language has
power, and moral language should not be applied to food.

Trash the restrictive patterns, too. You don't have to eat
a healthy breakfast. You don't have to eat any breakfast
at all if you don't want to. Or you can eat ice cream, if
that's what suits you. If you want to eat between meals,
you can eat between meals. You can also eat standing up

or in the car or both if you can manage it. None of these things is ''bad.''

Food is not a moral issue. It's just food. Embroider that on a sampler and put it up in your kitchen.

> ## FOOD IS NOT A MORAL ISSUE.
> ## IT'S JUST FOOD.

THE FAT BUDGET

The diet mentality will make you fat just as surely as it makes you unhappy. And reducing the fat in your diet in order to lower your setpoint can be approached as just another diet. What you really need is a pleasurable way of eating that (a) does not make you feel deprived and (b) has less fat in it. *The first condition is just as important as the second.* And it requires some knowledge and experimentation. You can't just assume you know which foods are low in fat and which aren't, for one very good reason. Almost everyone assumes that anything they like is high in fat and anything they don't like is low. It's not just ignorance that's the problem. It's *self-punishing* ignorance.

Try rating the following foods in terms of their fat content, lowest to highest.

1 flame-broiled Whopper

2 cups of pasta with marinara sauce

½ small avocado

2 slices of bacon, crisp

1 cup of Van Camp's pork and beans

1 milk chocolate bar (1.5 ounces)

2 tablespoons of vinegar and oil dressing

8 ounces of shrimp with cocktail sauce

1 tablespoon of tartar sauce

Did you feel confident that you knew what you were doing, or did some insecurities start to crop up right around the pork and beans and the chocolate bar? (The correct order is on the next page.)

Almost all of us can stand to take a good look at a nutritional guide, as well as at the labels of some of our favorite foods. There are hundreds of guides, available in any bookstore or library. We are not talking here about a calorie counter, mind. You need something that lists the grams of fat in each food and, preferably, other nutritional information such as sodium.

But there is another kind of information you need and, for this one, your only source is you. No biologist would try to categorize a new species without taking a close look at it. No artist would try to paint a still life with her back turned to it. If you are going to deal intelligently with your body, you have to take a long look at the life it's been leading.

To begin with, you have to know what you actually eat. This can be difficult for a lot of us. We've pretty much lost touch with reality where food is concerned—and we want to keep it that way. Some of us truly believe that we eat like horses, and we don't want to know what we are sure is going to be the ugly truth. Others are convinced that we're starving ourselves and, if we have to give up one more thing, we'll be living on air. The truth is almost always somewhere in between.

And the truth usually contains some serious surprises. For example, one woman lived on a quasi-vegetarian diet for years. She avoided fried foods, ate few sugary desserts, and assumed that her diet was healthy and low in fat. However, she ate a lot of nut butters, seeds, and cheese to provide protein. When she analyzed her eating, she discovered that, as far as weight control was concerned, she might as well have been chowing down on Big Macs.

Another woman felt guilt-ridden because she couldn't seem to get through the afternoon without a candy bar. It was the first thing she gave up when she went on a diet and it was usually the thing that ''broke her will'' and led her back down the primrose path. Looking at the rest of her usual eating patterns revealed that there were a lot of other foods she ate, foods that didn't really matter to her, that made the candy bar pale in comparison.

By the way, here's the correct order of those foods:

8 ounces of shrimp with cocktail sauce	0
1 cup of Van Camp's pork and beans	1.5
2 cups of pasta with marinara sauce	4
2 slices of bacon, crisp	8
1 tablespoon of tartar sauce	9
1 milk chocolate bar (1.5 ounces)	14
2 tablespoons of vinegar and oil dressing	16
½ small avocado	18
1 flame-broiled Whopper	36

So. You have to take a look at what you eat, how much, and when. The most effective way to do that is to keep some kind of journal.

Oh, my God, a journal!

Come on, you've made it this far. Don't leave us now. Not over a little old journal. Besides, you don't exactly have to keep a whole, entire journal. There are lots of different possibilities, depending on what you need and are able to keep track of. We'll give them to you in the appropriate chapters of this book. And these journals, inventories, diaries, notes, whatever you want to call them, are just suggestions. The important thing is to find a way to observe yourself. That's really all you're doing. You need to get to know your subject and so you have to observe it.

When you look over your journal, you're going to find out a lot about yourself. You'll discover not only your food choices, but your eating patterns. For example, there may be times during the day when you nibble endlessly. Or maybe your schedule creates long gaps between meals, much too long for you to be rational about food when you finally sit down to eat. Maybe, like a lot of busy people, you go through the day with no food satisfaction, even though you eat here and there. If you're in the habit of grabbing half a doughnut and a cup of coffee as you fly through the office or a handful of crackers and a diet pop out of your grocery bag, you may see dinner—your only real meal of the day—as an emotional and physical feast, absolutely loaded with food symbolism.

What the process of observation should do for you is provide you with a place to start when you're designing your program. What it should not do is provide you with fuel for self-condemnation. The way you eat is, may we reiterate, not good or bad. It is simply the way you eat. You need to know what it is so that you can preserve the parts of it you like, change the parts you don't like, and alter the things that are hurting you *without giving you satisfaction.*

Once you see what you really do, you will have the chance to make decisions about what you want to modify (or what you think you can modify without feeling deprived). But right now, understand that you can't look at any of this material through the eyes of the diet bullies. It doesn't matter whether Diet Workshop would frown on your having a salami sandwich for breakfast and pancakes at 9 P.M. for dinner. If that's the style and pattern you always go back to, why change it? Don't even consider any alteration that has failed several times in the past. If your lifetime pattern has been to be the last of the red hot cookie monsters, don't give a second's thought to total abstinence from sugar.

Your journal exists only to help you find options based on your own reality. If you can find the hidden fat in your diet, the stuff that doesn't matter, you can get rid of that and keep the cookies.

That's right. Keeping a journal may seem like a nuisance, but if you do it, you get to *keep the cookies.* Or the barbecued ribs. Or whatever it is that makes you happy.

You'll make changes, but they will be changes you can live with happily. And you'll make them very slowly. We have to say one more time that sudden, radical change is death to any weight control plan. *Never* overestimate what you can handle at any given time. Dieting has accustomed you to making superhuman demands on yourself. You expect to have to grit your teeth, bite the bullet, keep your chin up—why do all these endurance metaphors focus on your mouth?—and your expectations can sabotage you. Here's another one for the sampler.

> ## IT'S NOT A CHANGE UNLESS YOU LIKE IT.

What we're suggesting is much like making a budget. You use budgets for money and time because almost no one has unlimited resources. You spend what you can afford. When you blow your salary on a leather handbag, most people don't say, "What the hell, I might as well buy a fur coat to go with it." You can't do it, because you can't afford it. There's just not enough money in your budget.

It is amazing, though, that once people get tied into the diet mentality they don't see food that way. After eating a Milky Way, the average dieter may very well think, "Oh, what the hell, I've blown it. I might as well eat a chili cheese dog, a couple of orders of fries, and a chocolate shake."

Instead, try thinking of yourself as having a fat budget. There's a certain amount of fat you can "spend" in any given day. You may not have enough in the budget to afford both fettuccine Alfredo and banana cream pie, so you have to choose. This is not deprivation. It's common sense. It's also common sense to try an Alfredo recipe that's low in fat or a frozen yogurt banana pie so that you come as close to having both as you can.

> *TEN-MINUTE TRIM PASTA ALFREDO*
> *Make Lipton's Alfredo Noodles & Sauce*
> *using skim milk and replacing the*
> *butter with nonfat yogurt or nonfat*
> *sour cream. Sprinkle with lowfat grated*
> *Parmesan cheese.*

You can spend your budget any way you like. Suppose your budget allows for forty grams of fat a day. If you want to, you can use a chunk of it for a grilled cheese sandwich; you can "save up" for it by having cereal and skim milk for breakfast. Have a chocolate brownie using the part of your budget you saved by putting fat-free sour cream on your potato.

If you don't care what kind of dressing is on your salad, you can use fat-free and save the twelve grams of fat for a Milky Way. (Yes, a Milky Way is twelve grams of fat, and a dark chocolate Milky Way is only eight grams!) If you don't really care whether the pizza is double cheese and pepperoni with black olives, why order it? Get spinach with cheese and fresh tomatoes on a thick crust. It does make a difference.

When you make a fat budget, you decide in advance which of the foods your metabolism can probably handle without gaining weight. This is where knowledge about yourself is power. Figuring out what you really want to eat and organizing the possibilities is the kind of control you don't have in a diet program. If you are making advance decisions about what you will eat, it goes a long way toward eliminating guilt. It is one thing to run into the house agitated and upset and polish off the last of the Sara Lee coffee cake; it is quite another to plan to take a break in the afternoon for a pastry.

The next couple of pages will give you some numbers and information you need to work out your own fat budget. But first, let's look at journals.

You can start with a few notes. Something scribbled on

a deposit slip. That's where you make all your other notes, isn't it?

THE GREAT DEPOSIT SLIP FOOD JOURNAL

LIST CHECKS SINGLY	DOLLARS	CENTS
1 *FOOD & AMOUNT*	*FAT*	*CAL*
2 *Cheese Danish*		
3 *2 cups coffee*		
4 *2 handfuls M&Ms*		
5 *Greek salad w/Feta*		
6 *Dressing, 3 tbsp*		
7 *1 slice Vienna bread*		
8 *1 bag chips*		
9 *1 diet soda*		
10 *Oven-baked chicken*		
11 *Mashed potatoes*		
12 *Diet margarine*		
13 *Corn on the cob*		
14 *Diet margarine*		
15 *Carrot cake*		
16		
17		
18		
19		
TOTAL		

You can, of course, go on to another deposit slip. Your day's food intake need not be restricted to nineteen lines.

As you go through your day—or in the evening, while you can still remember—that's all you have to put down. Just what you eat and how much. Later, you'll get out your handy nutrition guide and fill in those last two columns like this:

LIST CHECKS SINGLY	DOLLARS	CENTS
1 *FOOD & AMOUNT*	*FAT*	*CAL*
2 *Cheese Danish*	8	130
3 *2 cups coffee*	0	0
4 *2 handfuls M&Ms*	7	155
5 *Greek salad w/Feta*	12	160
6 *Dressing, 3 tbsp*	18	180
7 *1 slice Vienna bread*	0	80
8 *1 bag chips*	20	300
9 *1 diet soda*	0	0
10 *Oven-baked chicken*	9	225
11 *Mashed potatoes*	0	150
12 *Diet margarine*	5	50
13 *Corn on the cob*	0	85
14 *Diet margarine*	5	50
15 *Carrot cake*	12	300
16		
17		
18		
19		
TOTAL	96	1780

You're probably going to be astounded at how few calories you actually eat . . . and how *much* fat. This is a very positive discovery. It means you are not going to have to starve to lose some weight. You're just going to have to make some cuts here and there in your fat intake.

If you're a little less resistant to journals and lists, you can keep your journal in a notebook and add a column for time of day.

The journal is the first step. Now, what do you do with it? You use it to help you keep inside your fat budget without feeling deprived.

THE SIZE OF YOUR BUDGET

We've said that you need to reduce the amount of fat in your diet, but how do you determine the right amount? There is no single answer. There are so many factors that affect how much fat your body can burn, you may arrive at the answer only by trial and error. Your gender, age, medical condition, and the amount of dieting you have already done are a few of the things working for or against you. Generally speaking, a woman who is over thirty and has done a lot of dieting will have to keep her fat calories at 20 percent or less of total calories in order to alter her setpoint. A man with the same background could probably go up to 25 percent.

How does this translate into food and calories? If you think that you average about 1,600 calories a day, you would try to consume only 20 percent of those calories— 320 of them—in fat. Since you are probably more familiar with fat in grams (as food is labeled), divide the calories by nine to see how many fat grams you can have in a day. (Nine is the number of calories in each gram of fat.)

---

1 fat gram = 9 calories
1600 x 20% = 320 calories' worth of fat
320 ÷ 9 = 35 grams of fat

There's a good chance you could stabilize, or even reduce, your weight if you do not average more than thirty-five grams of fat daily.

That's your budget.

But a word here about cutting fat. When everyone is screaming about lowering the fat in your diet, some of you may need the voice of reason to say some dietary fat is essential to good health. A deep cut in your percentage can only hurt you, especially if you are a woman who is still of childbearing age.

Fat is nature's way of ensuring fertility. Most women need some fat in their diet to have regular menstrual cycles. The production of estrogen, as well as other hormones, requires dietary fat. And a certain level of body fat—the amount varies with individuals—must be present before pregnancy can occur. Also, fat is your longest-lasting energy source. While carbohydrates are available to the muscle for quick energy, fat hangs around awhile and can be pulled from the fat cells when needed. Without dietary fats, your body cannot use certain vitamins, such as A, D, E, and K. There are also fatty acids necessary for building cell membranes. And you need a certain percentage of body fat to cushion vital organs and insulate you against cold.

What's more, fat has a big effect on the taste and satisfying quality of food. If you make drastic cuts in fat you are likely to be unsatisfied with your food.

So don't be a miser. Spend your budget.

SPENDING YOUR BUDGET

Assume that your budget is thirty-five grams of fat per day. Do you immediately cut your fat intake to that level?

Not on a bet.

That's the level you will eventually get down to. But if you try to take a shortcut and go there directly, you'll end up in Deprivation Diet Hell again. You can follow every single principle in this book, but if you don't do it gradually, you won't stay with it. And if you don't stay with it, your weight will go up again, *higher than it is now.*

No shortcuts. (Besides, sudden drastic fat cuts can be dangerous for those prone to gallbladder problems.)

Instead, you approach your goal with caution. Since you're probably up around eighty grams of fat right now, even a cut to sixty grams will begin the beneficial effects. Here's a step-by-step description of the procedure that we recommend.

1. *List your ten favorite foods.* Put them in order of importance. Really try to think about it. Even if you haven't had pork chops for years, if they're one of your favorite foods, put them down. Don't edit yourself for "moral correctness." If you actually love chili dogs, don't say that you prefer pasta primavera.

2. *Consult your nutrition guide and your journal.* If you can't bring yourself to keep a journal, you're now going to have to use your memory and be as honest as you can.

3. *Determine what you eat and when.* Go over a couple of weeks' worth of your journal entries. Look for foods that recur, that you eat regularly. Look for eating patterns. You want to base your budget on what you have actually been spending. Eating black olives on Thanksgiving, Christmas, and your birthday is completely unimportant. Nobody cares. The same goes for hamburger, fries, and beer once a month with your girlfriends.

4. *Look for high-fat foods.* Among those foods that you eat regularly, look for the ones that are high in fat. The others are basically irrelevant. Don't guess which ones are high fat and which ones aren't. Look them up in your nutrition guide.

5. *Compare your lists.* Once you have a pretty good list of high-fat foods that you eat on a fairly regular basis, compare that list with your ten favorite foods. Again, use your nutrition guide to find the fat content of your favorite foods.

If you follow these first five steps, you'll have a good idea of what you *want* to eat and what you actually *do* eat.

EVALUATING YOUR SPENDING

The next thing you need to do is use the information you've gathered to help you decide whether you're getting good value for your fat expenditure.

So, ask yourself the big questions.

- How many of your favorite foods do you *actually eat* regularly?
- How many of the foods you eat regularly are *higher in fat* than your favorite foods?

Those may be two of the most important questions you will ask yourself during this whole process. If your favorite food in the whole world is linguini carbonara and you *never* allow yourself to eat it, but you do eat tuna salad sandwiches from a restaurant near your office a couple of times a week, you are not doing yourself any favors. (Unless the restaurant has switched to low-fat mayonnaise, and most of them have not.) What you're spending on a discount store special would buy you a designer original. If you can replace some of the high-fat foods you usually eat with foods that are your favorites, you're ahead of the game, *even if you haven't yet reduced your fat content.*

Why? Because you're happier without spending any more. Remember, your satisfaction quotient is just as important as your fat quotient. So eat what you like.

Also, there may be foods on your favorite list that are very good expenditures in terms of fat. Eat them more often. Make them a larger part of your diet. Shrimp cocktail is a good example. It's a real favorite for a lot of people and it has *no fat.* If you go out to a fancy restaurant with friends and discover that the menu is geared to high-fat extravaganzas, don't order a salad. You'll look and feel pathetic unless you put on lots of dressing, in which case you might as well order filet mignon. Go to the top of the menu. Order black bean soup with sherry, Manhattan clam chowder, or French onion soup (sans crouton or cheese) for your appetizer and order shrimp cocktail as an entree. You probably won't feel the least bit deprived. But don't save it for an occasional treat. If you love it, have it for dinner a couple of times a month. Make it a staple.

OTHER GOOD BUYS

King crab with cocktail sauce	6 ounces	2 grams fat
Manhattan clam chowder	1 cup	2–3 grams fat
Gazpacho	1 cup	0–2 grams fat
Fig Newtons	1 cookie	1 gram fat
Pancakes (6-inch)	1 pancake	3 grams fat
Angel food cake	any amount	0 grams fat
Meringues	any amount	0 grams fat

MAKING CHANGES

The next step is to choose one *and only one* food that you think you could change. There are a couple of ways to make this choice.

1. *Start with something easy.* One possibility is to start with something really easy for you. Milk instead of cream in your coffee, as we mentioned before, might be one option, if you drink two or three cups a day. Low-fat mayonnaise on your sandwiches is another.

2. *Start with something for which substitutes are available.* Another choice might be something that appears on both your favorite list and your regularly eaten list *and* has some readily available substitutes. There are some foods that almost everybody likes

and that the food industry is working to make lower in fat. Take advantage of their labor.

Now, work with this one food until you've found a low-fat alternative or until you've decided that there isn't one. And then give yourself time to adjust. Until you do that, *don't try any more changes.*

For example, if you've discovered, by analyzing your lists, that cheese is an important part of your life, your job is to start trying low-fat cheeses, cheese spreads, and foods with cheese in them. Here are some of the options you might explore.

Low-Fat Cheeses
Of course, you can try different brands of low-fat cheese from your grocer's dairy case. Mozzarella is good, and so are some of the sharp Cheddars.

Low-Fat Cheese Spreads
You might get one of the fat-free cream cheeses and mix it with a sharp Cheddar spread. The strong flavor of the Cheddar will go a long way in combination with the bland but creamy low-fat cream cheese. Experiment with proportions and see if you like it.

An amazingly good option, if you like blue cheese, is a concoction that can be used as a spread, a dip, or a salad dressing. Blend until smooth low-fat or no-fat creamed cottage cheese, enough blue cheese for flavor, and a squeeze or two of lemon juice for extra tang. Again, experiment with the proportions. If you've been denying yourself blue cheese dressing for years, you're going to be happy as a pig in mud. (It's *a lot* better than bottled low-fat blue cheese dressings.)

Both fat-free cream cheese and blended low-fat cottage cheese are excellent bases for cheese spreads. Use your own imagination to flavor them, either with small portions of strongly flavored cheeses or with herbs and spices.

Cheesy Foods
Mix up a box of scalloped or au gratin potatoes, using skim milk and one tablespoon of low-fat margarine. You'll get the cheese taste and texture with a minimum of fat.

We could go on and on with suggestions, but you can probably find a lot of possibilities yourself by looking around at the grocery store. It's your job. And frankly, it's going to appeal to the bargain hunter in you. When you find or make a cheese spread that you really like that has only two grams of fat per ounce, it's like finding a box of Depression glass at a garage sale for five bucks. You'll probably go around telling all your friends and acting obnoxious.

Let us stress again that it's important that you work with only one item until you're comfortable or until you've given up. Then you can go on to another one.

ONE PERSON'S APPROACH

Take a look at the way Linda, one of Diane's clients, began working out her budget. First, she made a list of her ten favorite foods. It looked like this:

FOOD	FAT GRAMS	AMOUNTS
pepperoni pizza	6–30	1 or 2 slices, depending on brand
barbecued ribs	25	6 ounces of meat
chocolate ice cream	6–17	½ cup, depending on brand
french fries	10	20 fries
macaroni and cheese	10–30	1 cup, depending on brand or recipe
chocolate bar	14	1.5 ounces
french bread with butter	8	2 slices, 1 pat of butter each
hamburger	36	Whopper

cheese and crackers	15	1 ounce of Cheddar and six Ritz
muffins	1–15	1 muffin, depending on brand or recipe

She then looked over her journal for several weeks. It was obvious to her that there was a pattern to her eating. It looked a lot like the page printed below.

LINDA'S JOURNAL

TIME	FOOD	CALORIES	FAT GRAMS
7 a.m.	Two cups of black coffee	—	—
10 a.m.	Energy bar from the health food store	325	15
1 p.m.	Tuna sandwich and diet soda from cafeteria	400	14
5:30 p.m.	Small bag of chips in the car going home	200	12
6 p.m.	Batter-dipped shrimp from last night's Chinese food while fixing dinner	100	6
	Also while fixing dinner, two cookies and a couple of pieces of the kid's candy	160	10
7 p.m.	Meat loaf, dry baked potato, carrots, and peas	375	10
10 p.m.	Frozen yogurt	125	0
	TOTAL	1685	67
			x 9
			= 603

Linda's average daily food consumption is about 36 percent fat. That's not terrible compared to the average American diet. But it is still too high for Linda to maintain a weight of 145 pounds. This is partly because she is almost forty, comes from a family that is above average in weight, and has done a lot of dieting over the years.

Analyzing Linda's Eating Patterns

1. Linda doesn't have a lot of time for food preparation. She is a working mother with two children.

2. She tends to ignore eating during a large part of the day.

3. This leaves her ravenous by the time she leaves work.

4. She is hungry and stressed out by the time she hits home to prepare dinner, which is late because of her husband's schedule.

5. She fills up on whatever is available while making dinner.

6. The rest of the evening is very modest in amount and fat calories.

7. She thinks, as do many people, that anything that comes out of the health food store must be good for you. It might not be bad in terms of nutrition. However, someone with a weight problem needs to read the label carefully. There may be much better choices available.

8. On this particular day, she ate only one of her ten favorite foods (she considers frozen yogurt to be interchangeable with ice cream).

Because we included only one day of the journal here, there is another aspect to Linda's eating patterns that we have to describe to you. In the two weeks of entries, aside from frozen yogurt, most of Linda's favorite foods did not appear. She and her family did have pizza twice. On both occasions, Linda limited herself to one piece and tried to fill up with salad. And, on both occasions, she then ate at least one more piece cold the next day while fixing dinner. It's her favorite food, and she ate as much of it cold and left over as she did hot and wonderful. She never had french fries, macaroni and cheese (her husband does not consider it a "real" dinner), chocolate bars, hamburgers, cheese and crackers, or muffins. She also did not have barbecued spareribs. She no longer fixes them for her family because she loves them so much she's afraid she'll pig out. She had one piece of french bread with butter when she fixed spaghetti for her family.

In other words, Linda's food life is impoverished. She has robbed herself of pleasure over the years and now she has to get some of it back.

Linda's Changes

So, first, Linda looked to see if there were any high-fat foods she usually ate that she could replace with favorite foods. She spotted the energy bar from the health food store; she would be much happier with a muffin. To get a good, low-fat one, she decided to make a batch once every two weeks and freeze them. She takes one out of the freezer every morning, and it's thawed by her ten o'clock coffee break. This is a little more trouble than stocking up on energy bars and keeping them in her desk drawer, but she decides she can handle it. As a bonus, she saves almost twelve grams of fat! The biggest change Linda has made is taking the time to cook food she wants instead of eating food she can grab and store.

Next, Linda discovered the amount of fat in restaurant salad-type sandwiches when she checked them out on the nutrition counter. She actually would like a turkey or lean ham sandwich at least as well as tuna or egg salad, and the fat grams saved are probably eight to sixteen. If she really has a taste for tuna salad once in a while, it's not a problem. The rest of the time she is perfectly happy having lean cold cuts on rye with mustard.

So far, Linda has made two significant changes in her fat intake without any sacrifice or sense of deprivation. But the first one, at least, does require some effort on her part, so she decides to take a few weeks to see if these are changes she can live with.

There is one other pattern Linda has spotted that she would like to do something about. In an effort to diet, Linda takes great care to ignore her own needs when grocery shopping. Hence, when she gets home after work stressed, tired, and hungry, all there is in the house is "stuff she's got for everyone else." Her husband usually does not get home until seven for supper. That's a long wait, and Linda never prepares for it because she grew up with the diet philosophy of no snacking between meals.

This is completely unrealistic. If Linda accepts the fact that she is going to eat and buys what she wants, she will certainly do better than eating last night's batter-dipped shrimp and the kids' cookies. She is not going to make this a focus until she sees whether the other changes stick, but she does make the decision to try buying some new low-fat snacks and keeping them in the house all the time. If they work when she's hungry while fixing dinner, great. If not, she can always keep raiding the kids' cookies.

With just the two changes she has made, Linda has cut her daily fat intake by about nineteen grams.

blueberry muffin	3	health candy bar	15
turkey sandwich	3	tuna salad sandwich	10

After a couple of weeks, Linda goes through her diary again. There is one other small change she wants to try. She is hungry after work. She always thinks if she has some chips and diet pop on the way home, she won't snack so much before dinner. Most of the time it doesn't work that way. She's really hungry enough for dinner at six; a small bag of chips won't do it. Part of the problem is the need for a few minutes of rest and relaxation.

Linda's new plan is to try some other snack on the way home. She craves something salty and crunchy that she can chew. Pretzels are available in small bags in the commissary also. It's worth a try.

2-ounce bag pretzels	2	2-ounce bag chips	20

THE BEST PIZZA BUYS FOR YOUR FAT BUDGET
CHEESE PIZZA

BRAND	QUANTITY	FAT	PERCENTAGE OF CALORIES FROM FAT
GROCERY STORE			
Chef Boyardee Box Mix	*3.84 ounces*	*6 grams*	*24%*
Jeno's Pizza Rolls	*3 ounces*	*5 grams*	*23%*
Pappalo's	*1/5 pizza*	*8 grams*	*23%*
Tombstone Light (12-inch) (Veg)	*4.3 ounces*	*7 grams*	*27%*
Tony's French Bread	*5.5 ounces*	*8 grams*	*20%*
Weight Watchers	*6.03 ounces*	*7 grams*	*21%*
FAST FOOD			
Domino's (12-inch)	*2 slices*	*6 grams*	*16%*
Domino's (16-inch)	*2 slices*	*8 grams*	*18%*
Godfather's (Mini)	*1/2 pizza*	*8 grams*	*26%*
Godfather's (Small)	*1/6 pizza*	*7 grams*	*26%*
Godfather's (Large)	*1/10 pizza*	*8 grams*	*27%*
(Medium is higher in fat.)			
Little Caesar's Round (Medium)	*1 slice*	*5 grams*	*29%*
(Small and large are higher in fat.)			
Little Caesar's Square (all sizes)	*1 slice*	*6 grams*	*29%*
Shakey's Thick Crust	*1/10 pizza*	*5 grams*	*25%*

That's another eighteen grams of fat a day Linda has cut if she finds that pretzels do the trick. Two months later she has decided all three of her changes are permanent and her total savings in fat is thirty-seven grams per day. In the meantime, she's added several of her favorite foods to the list of those she eats regularly. For example, she's found a recipe for macaroni and cheese that is not absolutely loaded with fat. She now serves it regularly for dinner as a side dish and makes it her own main dish. She also eats two pieces when the family has pizza and then throws away the leftovers. *And* she eats french bread with diet margarine while she's fixing dinner at least once or twice a week.

Your own search for enjoyment and health in food may turn out very different from Linda's, but the possibilities are there for you. And when you discover the truth about pizza! Well, there's not much that can match the joy of finding out that there are lots of pizzas that have *less fat per slice than a tablespoon of vinegar and oil dressing.*

Ain't food grand.

> *The only way to get rid of temptation is to yield to it. Resist it, and your soul grows sick with longing for the things it has forbidden to itself.*
>
> OSCAR WILDE

SUGGESTIONS

1. Get together with a neighbor or two to make low-fat cooking a group project. You can trade recipes and new food finds.

2. You can also cook together. Three of you in the kitchen can make a vat of spaghetti sauce loaded with fresh basil, a half-dozen loaves of whole wheat bread so rich you could make a meal out of two slices, mounds of pasta salad, and a couple of batches of gooey low-fat brownies to be combined

later with chocolate frozen yogurt. You'll have much more fun than working alone and get more done.

3. Cook for your whole family the same way you do for yourself—healthier. You're not putting them on a diet, just giving them a new way of eating. And don't announce that the food you're giving them is low-fat. Just put it on the table.

4. Don't go to the grocery store without reading at least one new label. The fat variations between different brands of the same food can be remarkable.

5. Experiment making "mix" foods with reduced-fat ingredients. These include boxed scalloped potatoes, macaroni and cheese, pasta and sauce.

6. If you really like sweets, try hard caramel candies such as Sugar Daddies, Nips, or even Black Cows.

7. Plan a dinner of "memory" foods. Make a Jell-O mold, ambrosia salad, potato salad, or scalloped potatoes and whatever else makes you think of church socials and school picnics. Just leave out the meat.

8. Put together your discoveries in a pamphlet, sell it, and donate the money to charity. (See how much faith we have in your self-motivation?)

11

Skill Number Four:
Putting Your Life in Motion

Moving has nothing to do with whether or not I diet. It gives me a real sense of strength and control . . . that sometimes affects what I eat.

WORKSHOP MEMBER

AND NOW, ABOUT exercise.

Excuse me, I have to go empty the kitty litter box or something.

Stop right there.

No, really. There are calcium deposits around the faucets in my bathroom. I've just got to get rid of them.

You knew this was coming sometime. Just give us a minute. You don't have to join an aerobics class, buy an exercise bicycle, or take up jogging. You never have to darken the doors of a health club or pull on a spandex leotard. You do have to move. Increased body movement is a big part of both dealing with stress and enhancing your body's fat-burning potential. The more you move and build muscle, the more you reduce the percentage of fat in your body.

If you are a person who once thrived on volleyball and pickup softball games and have just let that go out of your life, your situation is, to say the least, enviable. You already like to move. Now all you have to do is work it back into your schedule. Find something you like to do with your body and do it. There are just a couple of things to keep in mind.

First, for weight loss, you need low-intensity exercise. Covert Bailey stresses that the best way to measure the intensity of your workout is your own perception. If you *feel* that you're working, you probably are. He suggests that you should be able to carry on a conversation while you exercise, but you should be breathing harder than usual. You should not be feeling the pain that comes with lactic acid buildup in your muscles.

Second, you need to get this exercise for about twenty minutes a day, three to four days a week. If you are trying to reverse the effects of years of dieting, more is better. Indeed, any movement is better. The same principles apply here as in dealing with food. *You* take control and you make choices that fit into your life. The thing to understand is that you can increase your activity without decreasing your enjoyment of your life even if your idea of the perfect evening is sitting in a recliner with a stack of mysteries on one side of you and a plate of pastries on the other.

WHERE EXERCISE RESISTANCE COMES FROM

If you are an exercise-resistant person, you have probably spent your entire life thinking of yourself as lazy. You've made jokes about how your idea of exercise is walking to the refrigerator to make another sandwich. When friends tried to get you into a volleyball game, you made noises about having a bad knee while, inside, you told yourself you were a sloth.

Sometimes, you read magazine articles that said you should always walk up one flight of stairs, do stomach exercises at your desk, and do leg lifts in your bath. It sounded like one hell of a good way to ruin your life.

What probably never occurred to you was that there

might be something other than laziness going on here. For a great many of us, exercise, especially sports and games, picked up a lot of negative associations early in life. This is particularly true of those who did not find social interaction comfortable or easy. What we say, and really believe, is that we don't like exercise or that we find it boring. What lies below the surface is that situations in which we engage in physical activity for its own sake are situations in which we expect to be inadequate and/or ostracized.

"When the teacher said we were going to play Red Rover, I used to feel my heart drop," says Hannah, a forty-six-year-old member of one of Diane's workshops. "I'd stand there on the playground praying maybe this time I'd be picked next to last instead of last."

The kid who gets picked last is a cliché of childhood. And, of course, we couldn't *all* have been picked last. However, if you were shy or a little different, if you just didn't feel as though you belonged, team sports brought it all to the surface. If you were fat, the situation was even worse. "I was afraid I'd do something stupid or clumsy and then everybody'd notice I was fat. I mean, they already knew, but I'd, like, call it to their attention," says Sophia, who has struggled with her weight all her life.

For those of us who are exercise-resistant, there are all kinds of negative feelings associated with sports, games, and other forms of physical activity. Just the sight of a volleyball net may be enough to make us break out in spots. These feelings are not always at the surface of our minds. For example, when you confront an exercise bicycle, you are not aware of any connection with rejection and isolation on the playground, but it's there. You don't expect anything with wheels and pedals to make you feel good; you do expect it to make you feel bad.

This makes sense. Children who find reading difficult seldom grow into adults who think of books as a source of pleasure.

This feeling is not helped when we put on workout leotards and see bulges everywhere. Those bulges are like signs we wear around our necks saying, "This body never climbed a rope, won a ribbon in a track meet, or got a hit in softball.''

If only you could tell by looking at someone that they can't play Scrabble.

Nobody is enthusiastic about activities that make them feel inferior. The world is full of people who never exercise their brains, but you can't tell that until you get them into a conversation. Those people react the same way when you suggest a party game like Password as *you* do when they suggest volleyball.

For those of us who feel the need to be perfect—a common need among lifetime dieters—the situation is even worse. We don't like to do anything we can't do well. We certainly don't want anyone to *see* us doing it, but we also simply get no pleasure out of doing things we're not good at. So if no one ever took you aside and *taught* you how to throw a ball, you probably don't like to do it. You feel your arm wrench half out of the socket when you throw and then watch the ball plop to the ground a few feet away. What's to like?

For those of us who are very large, there are some things we just can't do, no matter how hard we try. Our options are limited by the physical effort of moving a large body.

This is all exacerbated by our widely spaced and erratic attempts at exercise. Because of our unhappy associations with sports, most of us, when we try to increase our activity level, try ''exercise'' in its purer forms. We don't join a softball team; we jog. We buy a membership in a health club and try the stair machine. We do sit-ups on the living room floor.

And we hurt.

We almost always exercise above our fitness level, with the result that we experience the pain of exercise without ever discovering that it can feel good. We get bored with doing what is, essentially, a boring thing to do if you don't get to feel the physical exhilaration, and we quit.

The great thing and the hard thing is to
stick to things when you have outlived

the first interest, and not yet got the second which comes with a sort of mastery.

JANET ERSKINE STUART

And the next time we try to get ourselves to work out, we have even stronger negative feelings than before.

So, by this time, exercise means rejection, inadequacy, pain, and boredom. Who in their right mind *wouldn't* be resistant?

You have to get it out of your mind that what you're dealing with is laziness. If you're the kind of person who works sixty hours a week at your job or cleans and cooks for a family of five or makes three dozen macramé plant hangers for your church bazaar, you are not lazy. You have, however, lost faith in your body's ability to give you pleasure.

Questionnaire #5
Movement

1. As a child, were you near the last when teams were chosen?

2. How did you feel about gym class?

3. Did you find it difficult to join group activities at recess?

4. Did you feel that you could do physical things better when you were alone than when you were with others?

5. Was there anyone to teach you skills like throwing and catching a ball?

6. Can you remember a physical activity that you really liked? What was it?

7. Do you like to dance?

8. Do you give up on projects that require physical activity, such as cleaning your house?

9. Do you like to walk in beautiful places, such as on the beach or in a forest?

10. Does it make a difference to do something with a friend who you feel is your physical equal?

11. Have you ever used the time when you are walking, biking, or jogging alone for meditation or creative thinking?

12. How does music affect you?

What Do Your Answers Mean?
Do your answers generally indicate that you have unpleasant associations and difficult experiences with exercise? If so, look specifically at your more positive answers. For example, if you felt you ran faster when you were alone, or there is a physical activity you remember liking, you probably had a small, personal love for movement that was eroded by group experiences. That feeling of satisfaction with or even pride in your body was a private, very precious thing you held apart from the self-consciousness or embarrassment you felt in gym class. You may have protected it so well that, in your own mind, you don't call it exercise, won't allow it to be dealt with as exercise. There is a good chance that, given the right situation, you might be able to rediscover that feeling. The first step in the process is remembering.

> *Dance is the hidden language of the soul.*
>
> MARTHA GRAHAM

Maybe you answered question number six with a no. If so, think about it again. Close your eyes, if you need to, and try to remember the feeling of skipping with a friend, running in a new pair of tennis shoes, going barefoot in the grass, digging a hole in the backyard, or splashing in a swimming pool before you learned to swim. You may have to go that far back to remember a time when moving really made you happy. But somewhere back there, it did.

It can again, but you have to be careful. "My friend asked me to go out and walk on the track with her," says Tess, another workshop member. "I laid down the law right away. I told her I didn't want to walk fast. I didn't want to get out of breath. I would set the pace, and if she tried to make me go faster, I'd quit. I was defensive as hell, but I'd been through so many bad experiences with jogging and stuff like that.''

Tess was actually more than just defensive. She was downright hostile. It turns out, in retrospect, that she was protecting something that was important to her—the sense of competence that her body felt while walking. She wasn't going to let that activity be contaminated with the pain and shame of "exercise." Fortunately, her friend kindly went along with Tess's conditions. Now, Tess has two ways of walking—a slow, easy one for thinking and enjoying the view and a faster, more energetic one for feeling powerful and very physical—and they both feel good to her.

If you answered yes to the question about dancing, it's possible that you need some added stimulation to make exercise interesting enough for you. That's really true for most people, even those people who go out on baseball fields and "play ball." If you're not a ballplayer, you watch them standing out there in the outfield and you remember standing there yourself, bored out of your mind. Well, the truth is that the whole time they're out there, they're thinking fast and furious. What are they going to do if the ball comes their way at that particular moment? Where should they throw it? What runner will advance where? Who's coming up to bat next?

They're actually *interested* in the game.

A lot of that has to do with the fact that someone taught them how to play the game instead of just sticking them out in right field and telling them to catch the ball if it ever came their way.

At any rate, you can make sure that there is plenty of stimulation when you move. Hannah was so exercise-resistant that, having read Covert Bailey, she focused on stair-stepping as the most efficient way of getting in her exercise. She was converted to its necessity but she wanted to do as little as humanly possible. The book said that she could do stair-stepping for twelve minutes, whereas walking would be twenty. But Hannah discovered that twelve minutes of just stepping up and down seemed like an eternity. So she started doing it in front of the television during daily reruns of a sitcom she really enjoyed. She made a contract with herself that she could watch the show if, and only if, she spent the first twelve minutes stair-stepping.

It worked. And then an interesting thing happened. When she got to twelve minutes one day, she just kept going. Up to fifteen. Pretty soon, she was doing fifteen minutes most days, with twelve as a fallback position. Six months into the undertaking, she was doing twenty minutes most days. Then, one day, she turned on a tape of rock and roll instead of the television. By that time, she was involved enough in the movement itself that music was more compatible stimulation than television, at least on some days.

Hannah's progress has been gradual, and she will never be a workout fanatic, but her exercising has not involved shame or pain and it's been going on for a couple of years now. She will probably find that she can keep it up indefinitely. (And yes, her dress size has gone down.)

If you answered no to the question about giving up on housework, you have another insight into the way you operate. You're perfectly capable of sustained physical effort *if it has a purpose.* Games may not be for you. Jogging may not be for you. But cleaning up your children's playground every week with a group of volunteers could be right up your alley.

If you answered yes to this question, there may be something wrong. First, you need to have a physical examination to see if there is a systemic problem. Second, you need to look at whether you're providing your body with enough fuel. Keeping your body short on what it needs to move well is as self-defeating as things get in the weight control arena.

GETTING MOVING

Whatever you decide to do, start very slowly. Do not under any circumstances exercise above your level. If you have been inactive for a long time, that may mean that you start with ten minutes, or even five, instead of twenty. Fine. Any is better than none, and you will gradually increase your time. You may also start with something as basic as walking in place. Don't be embarrassed by that. Just do it. Your capability will change, and probably a lot more quickly than you think.

You need to think creatively about this question rather than just going out and buying a purple leotard and gritting your teeth. You don't want another exercise failure that will take you further and further away from a life with movement in it. Because movement is *most of the answer*. For everybody. It's most of the answer to accepting your body. And it's most of the answer to changing your setpoint. It's just plain most of the answer to controlling your weight.

Still, there is a chance that no argument we make is going to be powerful enough to get you started. That's the hardest part, getting started. It is also hard to keep going long enough to feel the reinforcement/reward that people find in moving their bodies. You have never experienced the relief. Maybe without a push you won't get that experience. So here's one last approach.

Try this. Go get a sheet of paper and a pencil. Sit down, somewhere where you can see a clock, and write a few paragraphs on the pain and chaos deprivational dieting has caused you. Put it down on paper, the worst stuff you can manage to write. Now, read it over. Think about it. Don't be ashamed of it, but remember how unhappy life has been for you.

Now stand up, right where you are. Start marching in place. Do it for a minute. For two minutes. As you march, *know* that you are moving way away from all that pain. Keep going for three minutes or four. For however long that sense of moving away from unhappiness will keep you going. Then stop and look at the clock. Whatever it says there is your first movement goal, whether it's three minutes or seven or twelve.

Tomorrow, of course, you'll make your situation more pleasant. When you stand up, you'll have the television on or the music playing. Keep moving just until you reach your goal, not a minute more. Do this at least four days out of your first week. In your second week, you can add a minute to your goal, two if you're feeling really frustrated. The same with the third week. In these first three weeks, you can do your movement more than once in a day if you want to, but don't do it for any longer than your goal. Ever.

And, every day, remember that you are marching away from pain.

After a few weeks, you can reevaluate your situation. You can choose a different kind of exercise or stick with marching but extend the time. You can add a stair-step. You can join a class or form an exercise group with other rank beginners. Do whatever you think you can stick with and enjoy. Learn to tap dance. Ride your bike to the park and back.

And if you find that you've made a choice you can't live with, go back to that chair. Don't scold yourself or be ashamed. Just think about what you want to leave behind. And start over again, *slowly.*

Whether you are exercise-resistant or not, pay attention to the other things that may be keeping you from doing this one thing that could change your life so much. You may want to begin your exercising alone, for example. When you feel your competency increasing, you can choose a more public arena, so long as it is a place where you're not going to feel judged. You also may have trouble with exercise that doesn't feel purposeful. If so, give yourself concrete goals. Don't just go out for a walk. Walk to the store to pick up something you want, to the dry cleaners or to the post office. That "place to go" may be just what your goal-oriented little heart demands.

So, be creative. And stop worrying about sweat.

Sweat? You think I worry about sweat?

We think that you worry about sweat, you worry about messing up your hair, you worry about finding time. Just watch.

If you want to incorporate movement into your everyday life, why not ride your bike to work?

I couldn't do that. I'd get all sweaty.

See? Now, the solution to this problem is simple. First, you shower and apply deodorant before you leave home. Second, you put on a T-shirt under your clothes. When you get to work, you go into the ladies' room, remove the T-shirt, reapply deodorant, and put your regular clothes back on. We asked several bicycle riders and they all told us the same thing. None of them has ever been accused of "not being fresh."

There's a similar solution to virtually every one of those distracting little issues about grooming and time.

"I used to call myself the only 150-pound ballerina," says Terry. "As long as I can remember, I've liked to move and dance. I love music. But as an adult it's a Catch-22. I'm forty-five and 40 pounds overweight, so I had problems going to the health clubs and the classes with the nineteen-year-old, 110-pound cheerleaders. And I don't like exercising alone. The stationary bike bores me to death. I know I'm not alone. A lot of women feel the same way. So we do nothing—except struggle over food."

But Terry *did* do something. "I asked two women in my apartment building if they would commit to a TV workout in my living room four days a week. I was shocked at how excited they were to try. Sometimes we don't fit in four workouts, but Monday, Wednesday, and Friday are solid. We feel good. We laugh together. To some extent I can say it's helped me to accept my body. You know, maybe I won't ever weigh less than 150. Maybe that will be all right."

Phyllis had to deal with several of these issues to make movement a significant part of her life. Phyllis was from a small town in the South. She was brought up to believe that grooming and appearance were a very important part of a woman's responsibility, to herself and to her husband and family. In order to live up to that responsibility, Phyllis had dieted for years. She never touched fried foods. She cut out sweets. She followed the rules in the women's magazines scrupulously. On a good day, she'd take in about 800 calories. On a bad day, over a thousand. On a "diet" day, she went down to 600.

Still, she was dissatisfied with her body. It was not the

size or shape she believed it should be and *could* be if she just tried a little harder to eat right.

> *The body is shaped, disciplined, honored, and in time, trusted.*
>
> MARTHA GRAHAM

Phyllis's break in this pattern came when she joined the YMCA because she'd just moved to a new city and was lonely. She went in the hopes of companionship. She started with swimming lessons. She had trouble at first, because swimming ruined her hairdo. But, for the first time in her life, she was feeling what it was like to enjoy what her body could do. So she changed her hair. Eventually, she came to care more about passing swimming tests than about the difference in measurement between her thigh and her ankle.

That's progress.

SUGGESTIONS

1. Call a friend you've been trying to make time to see, and invite him or her for a walk in the park instead of a drink.

2. If you have trouble getting started one day, or if you are getting a little discouraged, use any bribe or reward that fits into your financial picture. Promise to buy yourself a mystery or a lipstick or a bunch of daffodils if you finish your workout. If it will get you to move, it will be worth every penny.

3. Change your mental tapes. When you can't get started, trick yourself by saying, "Anyone can walk just one block." Promise yourself you can quit after the first block. If you decide to go farther, set another limit.

4. If the thought of other people watching you is unbearable, focus on anything you can do in the privacy of your own home.

5. Schedule your exercise in an appointment book, or make a contract with yourself.

6. If you can afford it, buy a treadmill. It will get around almost every objection you can come up with to exercise. If you want, put a sign on the display panel that says, "You are walking away from pain."

7. Choose a positive environment. Put an aerobics or walking group together yourself and include people you feel comfortable with. The group won't work so well if one person is a marathon runner, another is a twenty-year-old gymnast without a weight problem, a third is fifty-five and always dieting, and so forth.

8. The same holds true if you join a health facility. If you are forty-five, out of shape, and twenty-five pounds overweight, look for a place that makes you feel comfortable, where there are others like you. One of the big reasons people don't follow through at the gym is the feeling they don't measure up to everyone else. So, try the YMCA instead of a chic yuppie health club.

9. If you have the money, hire a personal trainer to come to your home. If you don't have much money, investigate what is available at the nearest branch of the "Y." Some now offer the services of a personal trainer for fees in the neighborhood of fifteen dollars a session. You might also pool your money with several friends to hire a trainer to come to one of your homes.

10. Choose clothing that you find comfortable and flattering.

11. If you work out at home, incorporate your equipment into your decor so that you don't have to get it out every time you exercise. Live with your stationary bicycle in the dining room unless company is coming. Use a low hassock for stair-

stepping instead of an ugly gray and pink plastic thing you'll want to keep hidden.

12. Invest in a headset and lots of tapes you like.

13. Find some people who play volleyball in the park or at the high school and rediscover your power serve.

14. Call your local branch of Habitat for Humanity and volunteer to help build houses for the disadvantaged.

15. Find out whether your local park needs coaches for softball, soccer, or tumbling.

12
Skill Number Five:
Moving Toward Something Better

❧

*There's got to be more to life than this.
I don't believe I was born to spend my
life worrying about my weight.*

WORKSHOP MEMBER

THE MOST IMPORTANT steps you can take toward controlling
your eating and your weight may have nothing to do with
food. Or exercise. Or even your body.

OPENING UP YOUR LIFE

Any psychologist knows that people with complex personalities and complex lives are much easier to help than
those who are focused solely on one area of human exis-
tence. If a person has a number of ways of defining herself
and supporting her self-esteem, she is significantly less
vulnerable to being devastated by difficulty or even failure,
which is usually limited to one of the many aspects of
her life.

> *Life engenders life. Energy creates en-
> ergy. It is by spending oneself that one
> becomes rich.*

SARAH BERNHARDT

In other words, if you see yourself as a mother, a lover, a bowler, a friend, a church leader, a gardener, and a potter, you're not going to be wiped out by rolling a 95 on your league night. Or drowning your new rosebush. Or gaining five pounds. You may be *really* unhappy, but you're not going to be wiped out. (If you think of yourself only as a bowler, that 95 is going to stay with you for months, haunting your dreams.)

Unfortunately, far too many people who have fallen into life-long dieting do not have this complexity of interests and self-definition to protect them. We have allowed the scale to become too important in determining what we think and feel about ourselves.

One problem here is that not only is obsessing unhealthy, it doesn't work. Fact.

> **People who worry less about their weight weigh less.**

That's not an easy thing to accept. Most of us have been brought up to think that, if you really work at something, you can achieve it. The diet centers play on this belief to convince you that, even if others have failed, you can succeed *if only you work hard enough.* But the relationship between your mind and your body is much more complex than Jenny seems to think. In this area, an effort of will can become a preoccupation that robs you of exactly what you need to gain control—happiness, satisfaction, fulfillment, adventure, excitement, and, ultimately, self-esteem.

However, as you have certainly discovered over the years, just deciding that you're going to stop being so concerned with your weight doesn't do diddly. What we're saying here is that you have to start worrying about other things. Redistribute the burden.

Open up your life.

*and he said: you pretty full of yourself
ain't chu / so she replied: show me someone not full of herself and i'll show you
a hungry person*

NIKKI GIOVANNI

After all, you have nothing to lose. If you go to Jenny Craig and are unable to get help for your long-term weight problem—which is by far the most likely outcome—you will have lost money, self-esteem, and a little more ground in the weight control battle. That's a loss. On the other hand, perhaps, even after you take up tutoring in an adult literacy program and experience the joy of opening up a new world to someone you grow to like and care about, you will still feel like a failure when you look at the scale. It could happen. But what have you lost? A little isolation, maybe. A little self-absorption. And you've gained the joy and feeling of usefulness. That's still real and still yours.

DEVELOPING WAYS TO COPE

Feeling a little lonely tonight? Well, of course you are. You don't really fit into any social group because of your size. Now, if you went on a diet and lost a little weight . . .

Feeling angry and frustrated? Someone else might think it was because your mother just ordered you to have your hair done before the family reunion, as if you were still fourteen. But you know that, deep down inside, she wouldn't care what your hair looked like if you were thin. Now, if you went on a diet and lost a little . . .

Feeling despondent, as though your life is going no-where? Things would be a lot different if you were thinner, more attractive. If you just went on a diet and lost . . .

*It's not the tragedies that kill us, it's
the messes.*

DOROTHY PARKER

If all you have ever done to get your life in order is diet, dieting is all you know how to do. You have not developed a repertoire of behaviors to deal with the issues that confront you from day to day. Of course, it's easier to take control of your food than to tell your boss you deserve a raise, your mother-in-law to mind her own business, or your best friend that she has hurt you deeply. But it doesn't *really work*. The problem isn't fixed.

There are other options besides food for coping with life. When you get that lonely feeling, you could try buying some clothes that you feel good in, signing up for a class that interests you, or joining a cycling club. They might be better ways to escape isolation than losing twenty pounds. If staying at home with your kids all day is your real problem, take them to a nature movie at a local museum. Or call your library to find out what programs are being offered.

Now, did you read the last paragraph waiting for us to get to the nitty gritty? If so, stop now. Why did you go blank on us? Why wouldn't you try some of these things?

For one thing, you don't really believe they will help. For another, you feel silly. Okay. But think about it. You've seriously considered having your jaw wired shut. Don't you think you can handle taking your kids to a movie on beaver dam construction in Wisconsin?

This is serious. Diet programs ask you to turn your life upside down, to make sacrifices and deny yourself. And, in a way, that may seem more appropriate to you. Your weight is a source of anguish to you, and we come along saying, "Why don't you try taking your kids to story time at the library?"

But the diet programs' drastic changes don't last. They don't go to the heart of the matter. And we're not pushing story time. We're pushing the idea that life is a big, complex, challenging endeavor. And if you confront its complex problems with only one arrow to your bow— manipulating your eating—it's not surprising that you suffer a lot of defeats. Or that, after a while, you begin to feel that your actions are futile. They are. You can't resolve the problem of loneliness in your life by denying yourself french fries. And so, eventually you feel powerless.

But you aren't powerless. It's *dieting* that's powerless. You have to understand and really believe that. Because your biggest obstacle to effective change will be the feeling that "Nothing helps. Nothing changes. Nothing works."

BEGINNING YOUR EXPLORATION

The point of all this is that you need to move *to* something better, not *away* from food. You need to find better ways to cope and more ways to enjoy your life. You need to develop the complexity of interests and values that will protect you and your psyche from devastation.

> *You need to move to something better, not away from food.*

How you accomplish that is between you and your imagination. Maybe it's trading baby-sitting time with a neighbor so you can do the books for the insurance agent down the street. You have to figure that out for yourself because we don't know that you took accounting classes in high school. This is your project, your job. However, this inventory may help. To see what sorts of things might go into a happy, satisfying life for you, note your feelings about the following:

Inventory #1
Life Enjoyment

1. I like being with groups of people.
   Very much ____ *Somewhat* ____ *Not at all* ____

2. I like spending time alone.
   Very much ____ *Somewhat* ____ *Not at all* ____

3. I enjoy activities in which I am a participant (games, dancing, sports).
   Very much ____ *Somewhat* ____ *Not at all* ____

4. I enjoy activities at which I am a spectator (movies, theater, sporting events).
   Very much ____ *Somewhat* ____ *Not at all* ____

5. Taking care of others gives me a sense of satisfaction.
   Very much ____ *Somewhat* ____ *Not at all* ____

6. I like to make things.
   Very much ____ *Somewhat* ____ *Not at all* ____

7. It's important to me to have intimate, not necessarily sexual, moments in my life.
   Very much ____ *Somewhat* ____ *Not at all* ____

8. I like to take risks.
   Very much ____ *Somewhat* ____ *Not at all* ____

9. Being with members of my extended family makes me happy.
   Very much ____ *Somewhat* ____ *Not at all* ____

10. Frequent physical contact makes me feel better.
    Very much ____ *Somewhat* ____ *Not at all* ____

11. I like to spend time outdoors.
    Very much ____ *Somewhat* ____ *Not at all* ____

12. I like getting to know new people.
    Very much ____ *Somewhat* ____ *Not at all* ____

13. Music makes me feel better.
    Very much ____ *Somewhat* ____ *Not at all* ____

14. I like to feel adventurous.
    Very much ____ *Somewhat* ____ *Not at all* ____

15. Solving problems gives me a sense of satisfaction.
    Very much ____ *Somewhat* ____ *Not at all* ____

16. I like personal conversations with people I know.
    Very much ____ *Somewhat* ____ *Not at all* ____

17. I like being the one in charge.
    Very much ____ *Somewhat* ____ *Not at all* ____

18. I like to feel that my actions improve the quality
of life for others.
Very much ____ *Somewhat* ____ *Not at all* ____

Look at the items you marked "Very much." They will
give you a sense of the things that you really need to be
satisfied with your life. Now, think about the degree to
which your needs are fulfilled in the life you're living
now. In fact, don't just think about it. Write it down. Look
at the last two weeks of your life and write down the
times when you met new people, felt adventurous, or enjoyed music, whatever you rated highly. Also write down
the things that you listed as not liking at all. How much
of your life is filled with those things?

For example, if you said that you like getting to know
new people very much, think about whether your life offers you the opportunity to do that. How often, in the last
two weeks, did you meet and get to talk with someone
new? If your answer is "not often," the next step is to
see whether that can be changed.

Could you get part-time work in a job that involves
dealing with the public, such as working in a store? Could
you volunteer time at a hospital or charity thrift shop?
Could you take a class?

The thing is, you have to start small. If your first attempt
to change the circumstances of your life is, for example,
quitting your job and trying to find a new one, you may
never try anything else again. Ever. You need some early
successes to build on. Maybe there's something you could
change about your situation at work. Something like moving your desk nearer to a window. Or asking for a new
software program you've read about. Any change is a start,
no matter how small. Next, try putting together a new job
resume. The mere act of responding to a couple of potential jobs is very empowering. You won't feel so much
frustration that requires food to relieve. Or perhaps you
could work with children with reading disabilities at your
local school and gain a lasting sense of satisfaction that
your job doesn't give you.

If you have trouble coming up with possibilities for

change, you may be unconsciously limiting your options. It's something we all do. Part of it's simply inertia. We resist change just for the sake of resisting. But part of it is the accumulation of beliefs that underlie our choices and decisions whether we know it or not. To see what beliefs may be shaping your life, note your feelings about the following:

Inventory #2
Life-Shaping Beliefs

1. By the time you reach a certain age, you should know what you want out of life.
   Strongly agree ____ *Agree* ____ *Disagree* ____ .

2. Most women need to be mothers to be completely fulfilled.
   Strongly agree ____ *Agree* ____ *Disagree* ____

3. I feel a strong sense of obligation to my parents.
   Strongly agree ____ *Agree* ____ *Disagree* ____

4. Most people who do odd or unusual things are just trying to get attention.
   Strongly agree ____ *Agree* ____ *Disagree* ____

5. If I don't take care of the people I love, nobody will.
   Strongly agree ____ *Agree* ____ *Disagree* ____

6. Doing more than people expect is the best way to keep a job.
   Strongly agree ____ *Agree* ____ *Disagree* ____

7. It's important to be able to get by without needing support from other people.
   Strongly agree ____ *Agree* ____ *Disagree* ____

8. People who hug and kiss each other in public are usually insincere.
   Strongly agree ____ *Agree* ____ *Disagree* ____

9. Being a good hostess is part of my job.
   Strongly agree ____ *Agree* ____ *Disagree* ____

10. Attention-getting clothing and behavior are in poor taste.
Strongly agree ____ *Agree* ____ *Disagree* ____

11. It's important to participate in one's extended family life.
Strongly agree ____ *Agree* ____ *Disagree* ____

12. There are certain material things, such as a house and a car, that any reasonably successful person should have.
Strongly agree ____ *Agree* ____ *Disagree* ____

13. There are few things more important than personal loyalty.
Strongly agree ____ *Agree* ____ *Disagree* ____

14. It's very important to be financially responsible.
Strongly agree ____ *Agree* ____ *Disagree* ____

15. People's actions should be guided by the rules of a higher power.
Strongly agree ____ *Agree* ____ *Disagree* ____

16. Being needed is more important than being wanted.
Strongly agree ____ *Agree* ____ *Disagree* ____

17. You shouldn't waste your education and training.
Strongly agree ____ *Agree* ____ *Disagree* ____

18. People who make a fuss over their pets are showing their emotional poverty.
Strongly agree ____ *Agree* ____ *Disagree* ____

19. It is better to give than to receive.
Strongly agree ____ *Agree* ____ *Disagree* ____

20. The respect of my community depends on my appearance and that of my home.
Strongly agree ____ *Agree* ____ *Disagree* ____

Let's look for a moment at how one of these beliefs could have kept one of Diane's workshop members from making a huge change for the better in her life. Cheryl is a teacher in her thirties. She was one of those women who worked all day and ate all night at home. Her job wasn't horrible, but it didn't make her particularly happy. It was just a way to make a living. It was stressful enough that, when she got home, she was too tired to go out and find ways to enjoy herself. So, she just sat in front of the television and did the one thing that she knew would make her happy. She ate.

Finally, Cheryl decided that her problem was serious enough to justify a radical change in her life. She quit her teaching job and took an evening shift working at a restaurant. Now, every morning from nine-thirty to eleven-fifteen, she goes to the YWCA. In the morning, she finds, exercise is easy and invigorating. She still has almost four hours before she leaves for work, but the exercise, she says, "has some kind of subliminal effect. I'm not likely to really pig out when I leave." For the rest of the day, she takes her energy with her to the park or home to do the laundry. The important thing for Cheryl is that her nonworking hours are no longer that time at the end of the day that she just has to tough out. They are the time at the beginning of the day that she enjoys and feels good about.

It was a big change to make and it took courage. But Cheryl desperately wanted to be happier and thinner. She's both.

Now, what if Cheryl had let #17, "You shouldn't waste your education and training" stand in her way? She'd still be standing in a classroom all day, using her education and being miserable.

> *There is only one success . . . to be able*
> *to spend your life in your own way . . .*

CHRISTOPHER MORLEY

Some of the beliefs you marked are firmly held convictions based on your own morality and experience of life. Those beliefs *should* be providing shape and substance to your life. But some others may simply have been handed down, without questioning, from your parents. Some may be prevailing beliefs in your community that you have adopted out of laziness. And some may be those of your spouse or your best friend. Those should *not* be shaping your life.

It is critically important for you to try to understand which parts of your life are of your own choosing and which merely a consequence of other people's expectations of you. A book that can be very useful in sorting out these issues is *Body Traps,* by Judith Rodin. In it, she deals with some of the ways our obsession with body issues reflects our social, cultural, and familial pressures.

SETTING LIMITS AND CREATING BOUNDARIES

At this point, many people ask, "But how can I make these changes with so many other people making demands on me?" All right, this is a big question, maybe bigger than you think.

There's a good chance that you are not a person who says no. You don't make demands yourself. These are things you don't like to do, things that make you very uncomfortable. In your mind, a good person's job is to love, nurture, support, and care for other people. In return, the other people are supposed to do the same for you.

Well, this is simply not true. A good person takes care of herself so other people won't have to. She makes her needs and desires known so that other people have half a chance of filling them.

> *Family is just accident. . . . They don't mean to get on your nerves. They don't even mean to be your family, they just are.*
>
> MARSHA NORMAN

She also sets limits about what is acceptable and what is not in her life so that she is not constantly filled with resentment over other people's actions. Limits can mean time and space, and you need both. If you don't have the time and space to meet your own needs—or if you think your needs are less important than everyone else's—you're in trouble. Because your needs don't disappear. They just get subversive. They go underground, looking for ways to get fulfilled.

Lorraine, for example, has primary responsibility for four children. Her eating was out of control until she inserted one more activity into her already enormously busy life. In one of Diane's weight control workshops, she heard the words "you are entitled to time for yourself," and they rang all sorts of bells. She read *Fat Is a Feminist Issue* and felt she really identified with "meeting everyone else's needs at the expense of my own. My husband isn't the least bit helpful either. He verbally sabotages any efforts outside of being a good wife and mother."

A musician since childhood, Lorraine decided to try out for the small local symphony in her suburb. She now plays with them regularly. As she has taken her music—and her right to make music—more seriously, she has broken away from most of her compulsive eating. But how does she find the time? "When I take myself seriously, I think my time at home practicing is more important than whether the laundry gets folded."

You probably don't have a flute to turn to, but there are things that can be changed in your life. There are ways to take control. You just have to be creative and remember that no change is too small, and no goal is too big. Think about what you might be able to do if you stop putting so much time and energy into controlling food and weight.

DEEPER ROOTS

Perhaps you feel your problems go beyond questions of job choice and talking to your mother-in-law. Perhaps there are deeper needs going unfulfilled or more serious emotional issues unaddressed. Maybe you feel that you are eating to escape from pains that go back into childhood and continue to affect you.

Using food to cope with pain or anxiety is really very normal behavior. It may have helped you get through some difficult times in a very difficult world. The situation becomes complicated when the eating begins to show. Now you have two problems, the unaddressed emotional issues and society's pressures to have a body that conforms to the ideal.

Dieting may help you combat the humiliation you have been made to feel about your weight. It may keep at bay the fear that you will just keep growing until you take up all available space in the known universe. It may help dispel fears that other things in your life are out of control. But it causes food to develop exaggerated importance for you while it creates a physical starvation response, and that is what can turn eating itself into something destructive.

A young actress, Janna, knew that part of what she was coping with was the sexual abuse she suffered as a child. During a visualizing exercise in Janna's workshop, she was the only one who could not remember a time when she was happy in her body. Not one time.

Janna made a major breakthrough in creating a new relationship with her body when she joined a theater group that performs in schools to inform children about sexual abuse. As she helped other children to understand and protect themselves, she felt stronger. She could not undo the acts that had caused her pain, but knowing that she was helping to prevent those acts from being committed against other children undid much of their damage. She shed her sense of herself as "victim" and her body as betrayer, and that was part of her process of freeing herself from food and weight.

You may not know what your eating and your body have been protecting you from. We recommend again that, in order to explore this aspect of your problem, you read *Fat Is a Feminist Issue*. In it, Susie Orbach provides a lot of exercises you can do that may help you understand just what you're trying to express through your body. These exercises are particularly useful in a support group. They can help break down shyness and self-consciousness and get you talking with each other.

For men, the Judith Rodin book *Body Traps* might be

more useful. It deals with many different roots of food obsession.

We do want to raise here the possibility that there may be very strong reasons for you *not* to want to open yourself up to change. Your battle with food may be, in part, a way of distracting yourself from other, more difficult battles. There may be some apparently irresolvable conflicts in your life. You might, for example, be dealing with the question of whether to put your mother in a nursing home. Or perhaps you know that your spouse is undermining your confidence and self-esteem, but you don't know how to fight that without leaving, which you are not going to do because you love him or her and have two small children. Or maybe you are bringing up your children in a dangerous neighborhood and can't find a way to get out. So long as you are angry with yourself about your eating, however, you can believe your major problem, your *real* problem, is food. And there's something to do about that.

Well, you may not be able to solve the central problem of your life, but you can almost certainly chip away at the edges of it. What's more, you can find better ways to cope. There are dozens, maybe hundreds of things you can do that no one else will ever realize are related to your weight battle. Some of them are listed below. The rest are hidden somewhere in your mind and in the world around you. If you're serious about confronting the issue of food and weight, you'll have to find them.

The important thing is to take your life into your own hands. Your first attempt may not be helpful, or it may not last. Weight control is a process, not a product (such as the number on the scale). It is trial and error. And error is not failure. In the diet programs, when you reject an option, you are considered to have failed. In this approach, finding that something doesn't work for you puts you one step closer to your goal.

SUGGESTIONS

1. Take a class. This one seems simple and dumb, but lives have been changed by classes. Just a couple

of years ago, a first novel was nominated for the National Book Award. Its author started writing when she took a class a few years earlier at a community college. And if you're single, you might be interested to know that more romances start in classes than in all the singles bars in town.

2. Teach a class. Chances are that you know how to do something that other people don't. Perhaps it's a skill that you take for granted, like sewing, arranging appetizer platters, or knowing how to look at a painting. Perhaps it's something you don't think of as a skill. Pam, for example, is a 200-pound woman who has never had trouble meeting and attracting men. She hasn't used that talent much lately because she is happily married with a couple of kids, but she still remembers. Recently, she advertised in the local paper as a counselor who specialized in improving "man-meeting" skills. One session and "results or your money back." Now she has two or three clients a week—and her methods work. (Which is neither here nor there, since that is not the province of this book. Maybe she'll write her own.)

3. Call your local park or community center to ask about classes for your children. While Johnny learns to swim, you can walk a few times around the track or just sit and watch your beautiful son get stronger and happier.

4. Volunteer. Choose something that's close to your own interests and/or fantasies. If you're stage-struck, for example, not-for-profit theaters always need help, whether they're amateur or professional.

5. Start a business. Okay, maybe just a small one.

6. Organize a "sewing circle." Our grandmothers had the right idea when six or seven women took their knitting, mending, or quilting over to the neighbor's for a couple of hours. While you're putting in a hem, you can catch up on gossip (or current

events if you're high-minded). Or you can take turns reading aloud.

7. Call a local museum and ask them to send you information about activities for children. Choose one that sounds interesting and put it on your calendar. Be sure to talk to your kids about it. Once they start looking forward to it, you're unlikely to back out. If you enjoy the first one, choose another.

8. Put a note on your door stating your schedule, times you want to be left alone to read or relax—the half-hour you want in the tub, the times you will be unavailable.

9. Announce at the dinner table how the kitchen will be set up, what foods are permitted in the house, what foods you prefer the family or your roommate to eat outside the house or keep out of your sight.

10. Let the kids know that, two evenings a week, they will have to get dinner started and set the table while you are at your aerobics class (or your bridge club or your painting class). Better to call a family meeting and decide on responsibilities than to sulk in the kitchen over coffee cake.

11. Let your husband grocery shop on Saturday so you have an hour to walk. Or go together, and walk for half an hour.

13
Skill Number Six: Getting Help

It seems to me that trying to live without friends is like milking a bear to get cream for your morning coffee. It is a whole lot of trouble, and then not worth much after you get it.

ZORA NEALE HURSTON

WE HAVE DISCOVERED that working alone on issues of weight is really doing things the hard way. You may want to consider either a support group or individual counseling.

In a society that consistently undermines attempts at self-acceptance, a support group can be a tremendously useful tool. It can also provide you with a safe place to be yourself. It will be easier to express yourself freely here than to people in your life, who may have a stake in your feelings and needs. If there are problems in your home life, you may not have the courage to talk to the people involved, not right away. A support group can help you think these problems through and, perhaps, come up with some solutions. Most important, a support group can encourage you to make changes.

*A friend can tell you things you don't
want to tell yourself.*

FRANCES WARD WELLER

Betsy, for example, had been going to one of Diane's workshops for some time without saying much; she was a very shy person. But something was happening inside as she listened to other women in the group and observed them encouraging one another.

At one session, she finally talked about her life. She was going to law school and holding down a full-time job, a job that was simply getting to be too much for her. It was draining her of the time and energy she needed to make it through school. (Her grades were low enough to put her on probation.) As she talked about the job, angry and frustrated with herself, it became clear that *no one* could handle what she was being asked to do, and the group told her so.

The next week, Betsy told the group that she had decided to leave the job.

Betsy had come into the group because she was so shy she felt that she had no friends and that she was isolated. And now, not only had she found the courage to change her life, but she had a whole group of people with whom to share her triumph.

(By the way, Betsy was replaced in her job by a man who is being paid more than she was and who has an assistant to help him do the job she used to do alone. She's contemplating a sex discrimination suit.)

Another option is individual counseling. Choosing this option does not mean you are "crazier" about food or weight than other people or that you have some deep-seated neurosis. A lifetime of dieting, deprivation, and strongly ingrained cultural beliefs about the female body may have established habits and patterns that require support and help to correct, that's all. If you have spent years dieting, eating erratically and secretly, and obsessing about the size and shape of your body, it could be difficult to modify your attitudes without professional intervention.

You may need a safe environment in which to risk giving up diets, a place in which to explore your real relationship to food and to understand what your body size means to you. You may also need help in finding alternative methods of coping with stress.

Questionnaire #6
Counseling and Support Groups

1. Are there problems in your life that you haven't talked to anyone about?

2. Can you hear advice about changing your life that makes sense to you and still feel hopeless about trying?

3. Does the idea of sitting down with a sympathetic person and talking about your feelings sound very good to you?

4. Are you seriously afraid of eating what you want when you want it?

5. Does your health insurance cover this kind of counseling?

6. Do you hide your eating?

7. Have you forgotten a time when you were happy and comfortable with your body?

8. During binges, do you ever become frightened?

9. Do you feel that your eating is completely out of control?

10. Do you have bulimic episodes?

What Do Your Answers Mean?
If you answered yes to all or most of the first four questions, you should probably try to find a support group where you can talk about your concerns and find the encouragement and understanding you need for this project. There are few reasons not to join a group and a lot of reasons to do it, so long as it is a group that focuses on

helping you with the three basic principles: taking control, making food a pleasure, and trusting your body.

FINDING A SUPPORT GROUP

So how do you find a support group? If you're a highly motivated person, you can start one yourself. If you have friends who share your concerns about weight, talk to them about the group, set a date and time, and ask them to invite others. An ideal group will have six to ten members, but you can start with fewer, hoping that your members will think of other possibilities as the weeks pass.

You can also ''advertise'' for members. Write a short notice explaining the purpose of the group and giving a phone number. Make copies of the notice and post it at your neighborhood grocery store, a local bookstore, the bulletin board at your church, your health club, or the YMCA. Use your imagination and you'll probably come up with other possibilities.

Your group should meet every week, at a regular time. There's nothing that will make a group fail more quickly than changing the day or the time every few weeks. Usually, it's best to meet at the homes of the different members, in rotation. That prevents the one person at whose home the meetings are held from becoming too central to the group, too much of a ''leader.'' However, if there are members who live at a distance or who for some reason don't want the meeting at their homes, exceptions should be made. Also, if a more public place is available, such as a room at a church, school, or YWCA, this can be the best solution.

We've already suggested that you use exercises from Susie Orbach's *Fat Is a Feminist Issue* in your support group. Reading aloud a few paragraphs from Geneen Roth's *Feeding the Hungry Heart* can be a good way to start a conversation, too. Or take one of the issues we've brought up in this book and start the ball rolling with that. After a while, you probably won't need discussion starters. You'll simply sit down and say, ''Tina, what's happening about . . . ?'' and you'll be off.

*Those whom we support hold us up in
life.*

MARIE VON EBNER-ESCHENBACH

If you don't feel you can start a group of your own, start
looking around. Try the YMCA or YWCA, local adult
education facilities, or the organizations listed in the
Appendix.

Women can look in the phone book under "Women."
There will probably be listings for everything from wom-
en's health clinics to women's bookstores to women's crisis lines. All of these are possible sources of information
about what's available in your area. You may feel strange
calling a bookstore to ask about a support group concerned
with weight, but the person on the other end of the line
will probably be, in addition to a bookseller, an active
member of the women's community in your area. She may
very well know a person or a group who can help you.

We *do not* recommend a group where there are weigh-
ins or where the entire focus of the group is discussing
weight and weight loss. You need to be able to deal with
issues in your life, as well as the emotions aroused by
trying to break your diet addiction. We *do* recommend a
group in which some attention is paid to the feminist issues surrounding weight.

The same can be said of an individual counselor. You
don't want someone who will weigh you, and you do
want someone who will recognize the social pressures and
family pathologies you are dealing with. If you answered
yes to the question about insurance, then there is no reason
you shouldn't at least talk to a counselor. (By the way,
most health insurance will cover this kind of counseling
if it is recommended by your doctor.) If you didn't, you
may still want to consider it. It will cost you less per week
than Jenny Craig or Nutri/System, if you take food cost
into consideration. If, however, money is a serious problem, look at the answers to the last four questions. If
they are yes, individual professional help may be important
enough to you that you want to call an organization con-

cerned with eating disorders and ask about publicly funded programs or counselors with sliding scales.

Looking for the help you need is part of your project. You should be careful, of course, to find people who are interested, not in controlling you, but in helping you gain control for yourself.

EVALUATING A COUNSELOR

What kind of help is available? How do you go about finding and evaluating a counselor? Ideally you might get a personal recommendation. Make sure the person is not a "kindly M.D." or a psychologist seen by a friend for marital counseling. You need someone with special training.

If you do not have a personal recommendation, there are at least four organizations you could contact. They are listed, with their addresses, in the Appendix. There is also a national newsletter, "Eating Disorders Digest," published in Baton Rouge, Louisiana. For information, look at Resources in the Appendix.

Even after you have a local contact for a counselor or a group it is still scary to start therapy. How will you know if the person you are dealing with is any good? There are bound to be some uncomfortable feelings, some conflicts and tension in the discovery process. But as the book *Surviving an Eating Disorder,* by Michele Siegel, Judith Brisman, and Margot Weinshel points out, there is such a thing as a good match between client and counselor. The basis is trust. How do you feel about being open, honest, and vulnerable with this person? In order to grow, to heal, and to move forward, you need an environment safe enough to reveal yourself. You need an atmosphere of unconditional acceptance. This is the seed of self-acceptance, and, as we have pointed out, self-acceptance is the beginning of everything. Trust your instincts. Don't be afraid to interview several counselors before making a decision. Do not hesitate to terminate counseling if you feel "the match" just isn't working.

If you're uncomfortable just going in cold, if you're afraid you won't know how to figure out whether the counselor is right for you, here are some questions you might ask and some hints of what to look for in the responses.

1. *What do you think causes people to be overweight?*
   You're looking for someone with a balanced view. Does the counselor mention physical as well as emotional factors? Do you get any sense that the counselor sees the issue as a problem in our society as well as in your life?

2. *What is your approach to the problem of overweight?*
   You need help with your life. Are you going to get it, or are you going to focus entirely on your size? Does the counselor mention exercise or increasing your physical activity? Is dieting recommended?

3. *How would you define overweight, compulsive eating, an eating disorder?*
   You can tell a lot by listening to someone talk about what being overweight is. Anyone who refers to charts is probably on the wrong track. Someone who uses terms such as "compulsive eating" as though they have clear, unquestionable definitions may also be more limiting than you want.

4. *What's your success rate?*
   This can be a real eye-opener. If the counselor starts talking about how many of his or her patients have lost what amounts of weight, get out of there.

Talking with the counselor about these issues will also give you a chance to sense whether there is a personality match. If you don't like the *person*, you won't get much help from the *professional*.

There is no special magic the counselor has. Progress is the result of your working hard together. A good counselor will not begin with a preconceived agenda, but will be the first to agree that no one knows you better than you know yourself. He or she will take clues from you and build on your strengths first

14
When You've Lost Touch with Hunger, Food, and Feelings

❧

*I like feeling hungry. I know it represents
power and control. When my stomach is
full, I feel awful, out of control of my
body and my life. I don't like myself*

DIET PROGRAM CLIENT

DIETING CAN GET out of control.

That may not be the way you think of what has happened in your life. You may think that it's your eating that's out of control or perhaps yourself. But there's really no question anymore about this particular chicken and egg. If you started dieting at an early age, and your diet history is extreme in kind or in length, that dieting has almost certainly caused serious problems with food, perhaps significantly more serious than any we've talked about so far. If so, these next three chapters are designed to help you deal with the destructiveness you've experienced.

*Hope is the feeling you have that the
feeling you have isn't permanent.*

JEAN KERR

THE DESTRUCTIVENESS OF DIETING

The sad fact is that approximately two thirds of all diet program clients have subclinical eating disorders. They are caught in a spiral of starvation and bingeing, of iron control and terrifying lack of control. No diet center can help you deal with these feelings and no diet center can give you the tools you need to rebuild a healthy relationship with food and eating. They don't acknowledge that the problems exist and they certainly don't have the sophistication to address them.

For some of us, dieting has been easier than the pain we've used it to escape. Because we've also gone through some personally proportioned mixture of these elements: self-directed anger, basement-level self-esteem, loss of confidence, humiliation, social prejudice, isolation, and ridicule.

If this is your experience, you may be skeptical about advice. With good reason. There are a lot of people out there telling you what to do who don't know what you've been through and don't know what you feel. While we're not going to say that no one can understand these issues who hasn't lived them, we have found that firsthand experience is extremely useful when it comes to addressing the problems of the lifetime dieter, for whom the emotional and the physical are so intertwined. For that reason, it may be useful for you to know Diane's background.

Diane's Story

I am an artist, a therapist and a sometime writer, would-be actress, and former teacher. I say all these things with pride.

I am also a person who has struggled with weight and diets all of my life. I have been almost anywhere the food/weight obsession can take you. That I say with a mixture of pain and strength.

I was a very average chubby kid. I mean average in appearance, but rounder by age eight or nine. By the time I was eight I did not want anyone to take my picture. It came to my attention that my appearance had flaws. Something needed fixing. My body was not so different from that of other girls, a bit too round and full. By age twelve, I had hit my peak of 148 pounds. My body, which I previously thought was my business, became the subject of comment. I became the object of "well-meaning" remarks. "It's amazing Diane dances so gracefully, considering her size." I stopped dancing in front of other people.

My family and other significant people did not think I was average enough. They focused on my weight. My body had become too big and unacceptable. That is what I saw reflected in my family mirror. I did not resemble my lanky, thin cousins or playmates.

"Diane, you'd be so pretty if you just lost some weight!"

"Diane, you can stand up for cousin Ellen's wedding if you lose twenty pounds."

"Diane, if you lose a little weight, you can take modeling lessons. We'll get you new clothes. Anything for you, Diane, if you lose weight."

"Diane, no one will marry a fat girl!"

These are the bits, pieces, and sentences that are locked in the recesses of my mind. They are the threads and fiber of my dreams and my nightmares. It did not take long for me to understand that to be thin equaled happiness, love, and power. These things I longed for and felt denied.

I retaliated with eccentricity and a drive for perfection. I was going to be the best, the smartest, and one of the world's most fanatic overachievers. Only perfect was good enough.

As I said, by the time I was twelve I weighed about 148 pounds. The school nurse, to my chagrin, made a public announcement to the class. (All of whom, no doubt, had the course of their lives changed by this revelation.) As a result, my mother took me to the doctor. I was desperate to please, to be acceptable. She must have felt desperate about the state of my appearance. I feel this is true, but I also know that this was done out of ignorance. It was a common phenomenon in the culture and time of my adolescence.

I eagerly accepted when the family doctor gave me diet

pills and a 1,200-calorie diet. Initially I lost about twenty-five pounds. Then the diet was quickly abandoned, but the diet pills hung on, off and on, for another twenty-five years. Even when I wasn't losing weight, I could do almost superhuman feats on the stuff—clean the house in five minutes flat, walk the dog to Canada and back and paint a pointillist masterpiece when I returned.

If I was not the type who pushes life to the limits, I might not have gotten into a barrel of trouble. On the other hand, I might still be another unhappy "round-looking woman" looking for the next diet. That is not something I can analyze; it's me.

I started out dieting like all the women around me. Every cockamamie diet that came out. If I was too fat, it was morally correct for me to have a Metrecal shake (a relic of the sixties, now marketed in the form of Slim-Fast) for dinner, while everyone else ate food. Unless you are reading this book for a lark, and that's unlikely, you are fully aware of the tyranny of the scale, the tyranny of the diet, and the tyranny of the world around you that WATCHES! all the things that rob you of life. Two "new" pounds could create havoc in my day. A half a box of cookies could put me in a tailspin for a week.

The dieting escalated, became more rigid and bizarre. Eventually, my life was about weight and dieting. And then I just stopped eating. Diets didn't work anymore, and emotionally I couldn't deal with diet deprivation. It was easier to do without entirely.

At thirty, I found myself in a psychiatric ward, dying of malnutrition. I am one of the lucky ones, I am still around to tell this story.

On reflection, the most painful part of my story was not being in a locked ward. Maybe I had to get to that point to start over. The worst was realizing that I lived, and live, in a world that fosters this insanity as "right thinking." A life that revolves around a number on a scale and the calories in a slice of melon.

It wasn't just that I weighed ninety pounds. The irony was that now I was thin, beyond perfection, and I was unhappier than I'd ever been. A devastating insight. Being thin had not brought any of the dreams my family and the world had promised. But I didn't know how to stop. I could never be fat, even chubby again. Not all of us change gracefully. Some of us, eventually and reluctantly, manage to change with tremendous clumsiness. My recovery from compulsive eating and starvation was not a straight line. The first step out was realizing I needed help, and not diet help. But, like all human beings, I made some wrong turns, fell all over myself, and blundered around in circles. Learning is not neat.

I could not have handled this battle alone. This is not an admission of weakness or wisdom. Just a fact. I must have been in the right place at the right time. In the hospital, a young (new on the staff) therapist was assigned to me. He was a maverick. He arrived at our first appointment in cowboy boots. He appeared without an agenda or any preconceived notions of how to "change" me. He refused to judge all the things I'd come to judge about myself.

I resisted this madness at first. Couldn't he see I was hopeless? But my ravings were met with a simple, "How can I help you?" I would rail about my bingeing and bizarre eating habits. I would cry, "When will this end, when will I give up this crazy behavior?" He would respond, "When you are ready."

What he meant was, when this ritual no longer has any value to you, you'll put it aside. When food and denial of food are not necessary for survival, they will go. When you are not so frightened anymore, you can let go and take risks. You need alternatives and options to make a trade. Then it will not be a matter of giving anything up. You will move on.

He was right.

And then, for the first time in more than a year, the hunger came back. The one thing being anorectic had allowed me to escape was the insidious hunger, the hunger that drove me mad every time I put a bite of food in my mouth. It was the great seduction of anorexia—freedom from hunger. When it returned, it returned with a vengeance.

The hunger never let up, from the moment I woke up until I went to sleep . . . then all through the night. I rose from sleep to eat often during the night. Anything. I found debris in the morning that looked like the remains of a drunken spree. I could never fill the hunger. Deprivation that spanned months, years, the better part of my life, appeared to have left me constantly needy for food. The fact that I had believed dieting was the answer to life had created insatiable hunger. It had also distracted me from finding options, other avenues to fill the hunger. During these years I did not paint or write or dance—I just dieted.

It was a slow beginning. I had to sort out the personal meaning of happiness and freedom from the arbitrary standards I had imposed on myself; I had been living as if a perfect body were happiness. It took me a long time. But the point is, with help, I got there.

During this same time, I finished graduate school and started my own part-time counseling practice in eating disorders. It was not an easy decision, knowing I still had a distance to travel myself. It proved, however, to be the right decision for me. I also began to study with a New England artist who has been my friend and mentor for eighteen years. I met Kathleen, who also became my friend, confidante, and touchstone with feminist thinking. Something was developing that had been truncated many years ago, lost in years of diets and anorexia. Self-esteem. Indeed, I was not crazy.

There were other significant events that created the change. Part of my healing has come from the creative work I do, my solid image of myself as an artist, a maker of beauty. Whether I weigh 100, 150, or 200 pounds, I think of myself as a maker of beauty.

I discovered that the process of coming to terms with food and your body has nothing to do with denial and walking away from food. It has to do with walking toward something better.

Long before I turned fifty, I knew I had been hauling chapters of this book around in my head for a very long time. At fifty, I have more weight around my middle than Dixie Carter and I still feel qualified to write it. I do not look like a model, yet I would not shy away from posing for the book cover. (It's simply that no one asked.) I'm just okay. I don't claim to have perfected anything. I'm not a "finished piece." I am a survivor. I have come to truly like my flaws, quirks, and imperfections.

Being a survivor is a process of self-discovery. I don't say I have the whole act together, but it's looking a lot better. I am still the product of a culture and a family that believes overweight is bad, fat people should be dieting, always, and your body is never good enough. Thirty years ago, I bought all this. A lot happens in thirty years. And I'm delighted to return the goods.

Milestones and personal victories. I threw out my scale twelve years ago and I still know who I am. I eat in restaurants now, and in front of other people. And I wear red.

My journey is not over, far from it. But I know that anything is possible! That includes throwing out the scale, ignoring *Vogue* magazine, and telling the doctors you don't want them to weigh you. It includes sending a painting to a show in Paris and writing a book.

Oh yes, and eating chocolate in public.

WHEN FOOD AND HUNGER DIVORCE

Dieting is *designed* to pervert all your body's natural instincts about food. Every rule is created to deny hunger and every guideline to stifle your body's need for nourishment.

When you're on a diet, "hungry" is irrelevant. If you follow this kind of plan often and long enough, your body doesn't know what you're doing. And you sure don't know what it's doing. When hunger becomes divorced from food, food becomes divorced from hunger. When you don't eat when you're hungry, you eat when you're not hungry. "Diets teach people to ignore the natural biological signals of hunger and satiety," says Dr. Janet Polivy of the University of Toronto. "Then when they go off the diet they don't know when to stop eating."

Hunger does not breed reform; it breeds
madness and all the ugly distempers that
make an ordered life impossible.

WOODROW WILSON

"I don't know why," says Dana, a mother of three whose eating problems began in an abusive marriage and continued through both Nutri/System and Jenny Craig, "but I vaguely remember, when I was a kid, food was just food to me. If I was hungry, I ate, but it didn't 'call to me' the way it does now."

"I really don't know hunger," says Brenda, a school-teacher who has been on Nutri/System on and off for years. "I mean I see cookies, I just have to eat them. I don't remember even enjoying food lately. I sometimes keep searching for one more thing that will hit the spot. By then I've had a whopping binge. Am I hungry ... or crazy?"

Your relationship with food may not be as extreme as Brenda's, or it may be worse. If you're a dieter at all, you've probably felt "food mad" at least when you were in the middle of a diet. Once you were eating again, it went away and you didn't worry about it. If it has become a part of your life, however, you probably think it's a result of some emotional problem. Even if no one has ever said your food behavior was crazy, it *feels* crazy to you.

"At one point I actually chained the cabinets at night," says Margaret, a former diet pill addict, "and gave my husband the key. I felt like part of an 'I Love Lucy' show, but if there was something good in the house I'd wake up during the night and finish it off."

Now we know that one of the major reasons Margaret was driven to falling on a bag of potato chips like a starving wolf is that food developed a symbolic power for her while she was dieting. (Another reason is that she actually *was* starving. Remember the starvation response to dieting?) When food is the one thing you deny yourself, it comes to seem that it is the only thing you need.

There's only one way out of this trap. You have to start trusting your body's need for food again.

RECOGNIZING HUNGER

The first step in getting uncontrolled eating under control is to learn to feel when you are hungry and feed yourself when and what you want to eat. This valuable insight is explored in depth in the book *Overcoming Overeating* by Jane R. Hirschmann and Carol H. Munter, and, if you are a person whose years of dieting have resulted in serious compulsive eating, you might very well want to take a look at it. (For information about the book, see Resources in the Appendix.)

However, to go directly from counting every calorie to "adult feeding on demand"—the method recommended by Hirschmann and Munter—is a gargantuan leap for people who have been dieting for a long time. The feeding on demand approach requires that you attempt to eliminate all eating that is not inspired by physical hunger; that you eat every time you get hungry and that you eat, as nearly as possible, exactly what you want to eat; and that you never eat when you are not hungry or what you are not hungry for.

While we agree with the concept of nurturing your body in a way that suits you, we think there are some steps that can make it a more gradual process, things you can do along the way to give yourself the support and courage you need.

We also think that eliminating all eating except that which is inspired by physical hunger is not the ideal state. It may be, for some longtime compulsive eaters, a situation that must be accepted. But it is not ideal. The ideal situation includes eating cake at your child's birthday party and a hot dog at a ball game.

To reach that goal, you have to stop thinking of your body and its urges as your enemy. Restricted eaters are compulsive eaters. Period.

This will be difficult, but it can be done. To begin the process, you must distinguish between hunger and nonhunger eating. You want to feed your hunger and eventually *moderate*, not eliminate, your nonhunger eating. And until you eat when you're hungry, you won't be able to figure out the difference.

To begin with, for a while, we want you to rate your level of hunger and fullness each time you eat. The inability to recognize hunger is as dangerous as the inability to recognize pain. Think of this as developing another survival skill.[1]

First make up a rating system to define hunger and fullness. Let's say you use the numbers 1 to 10; 1 represents that feeling you have when you have gone beyond hungry to sick. You feel weak, headachy, and faint. You probably have skipped at least one meal. At 2, you are ravenous, ready to eat the dog when you come through the door. At 3, you are moderately hungry and could easily eat a good meal. At 4, a snack will take care of any hunger you have. Five is the middle point. It's sort of the way you feel after you've had a snack. You're not hungry, but you're not really full, either.

Now we're rating your fullness. At 6, you've finished eating and you're satisfied, but there's always room for dessert. At 7, you're full, but not uncomfortable. By 8, you are stuffed. At 9, all you can do is stagger over to the sofa and lie down. At 10, you're sick.

If you start the diary and have trouble rating your fullness, you might try this exercise. While you are learning, try to eat without distractions. After several bites, put your fork down, close your eyes, and put your hands on your stomach. What does it feel like? Eat a little more, and do the same thing. At some point, you are likely to feel physically satisfied in a way that you can identify, even though you continue to eat afterward. At this stage in the process, don't try to make yourself stop eating when you feel that

---

1. You will find a variety of suggestions for discovering these two feelings in Judy Wardell's book *Thin Within*. Most of the book is devoted to finding out about yourself. The exercises that follow are of the type that she developed.

"click." Just use it as a way to measure your fullness. It's obvious that this is not an experiment to do when you are on the freeway going sixty miles an hour and trying to stuff down Chicken McNuggets before your two o'clock meeting. It probably won't work when the kids are in the kitchen nagging you about dinner and help with their algebra homework. But when you can use it, try it.

Now, you're going to use this rating system to keep a diary of your hunger and fullness.

DIARY #1
HUNGER/FULLNESS

TIME	FOOD	AMOUNT	HUNGER LEVEL	FULLNESS LEVEL

What Does Your Diary Say about Your Eating?
This is a consciousness-raising exercise. It is intended to help you find out and make yourself aware of your eating patterns. Many longtime dieters will tell you their eating is completely emotional. If you are one of these people, this is your chance to figure out whether that is really true.

Look at the numbers in your hunger-level column. How often do you eat at 1 or 2? If it's often, what you think is binge eating may actually be just feeding extreme hunger.

But how do you get that hungry? Look at the time, food, and amount columns. Are you waiting more than four hours to eat? During the day do you grab an apple and call it lunch? Maybe your food isn't stretching far enough for your hunger.

We need to add a little to your knowledge about metabolism here. Carbohydrates are digested, meaning used up, in a couple of hours. Refined carbohydrates go even more quickly. So if all you had for a meal was fruit or toast, chances are you will be hungry, really hungry, after a couple of hours. If you have candy you may be hungry as little as an hour later, unless it's candy that has significant fat, such as chocolate.

Protein foods last a little longer than carbohydrates, depending on the amount of fat in them. For instance, nonfat yogurt might hold you for three hours, while a chicken breast will last longer. Fat, on the other hand, stays with you for about seven hours . . . or forever, if you can't burn it off.

DIGESTION TIMES
FOR DIFFERENT
FOOD TYPES

Refined carbohydrates	*about an hour*
Complex carbohydrates	*a couple of hours*
Protein without fat	*3 or 4 hours*
Protein with fat	*4 or 5 hours*
Fat	*about 7 hours*

If you are already following the current trends toward high carbs and low fat, you really do need something to eat every few hours during the day. And, if you follow classic dieter patterns, which is to exist on air until three in the afternoon, your afternoon and evening binges are predictable.

So go back to your inventory and take a more sophisticated look. Look at the type of food you're eating. If you are waiting too long, eating too little sometimes, and virtually avoiding protein and fat most of the day, it's no wonder your food isn't stretching to meet your needs. You may be doing nothing wrong except ignoring the reality

that your body needs more food or a little protein during
the day.

Now look at your fullness numbers. If they are consistently 8 or over when you have stopped eating dinner, you
are probably looking at the result of the pattern we just
talked about. If you go without food for seven or eight
hours and work out at the gym on your way home, you
should not be surprised that your body demands a bucket
of Kentucky Fried Chicken, a half-dozen rolls, and a bowl
of mashed potatoes. You are so ravenous you leave yourself no choices. Besides overeating, you are probably
eating anything you can get your hands on. You are not
able to control either the quantity or the type of food you
eat, and that lack of control is tied into this pattern, *not
to emotional hunger.*

You need some pacing.

FOOD AND FEELINGS

Or maybe you discovered a different pattern when you
looked at the numbers. Perhaps you eat constantly. You
have bits of this and that, things that look good or are just
offered to you, even when your hunger level is 4 or 5.
One possible explanation for this is that you never go long
enough to allow yourself to feel hunger. You handle general anxiety with food.

Another possible explanation for the same kind of eating
pattern is that years of denial and dieting have caused you
to fear hunger in general and avoid it at all costs.

Or, you may have specific connections between particular emotions and eating.

If you keep the hungry/full inventory for a few weeks,
patterns will emerge that you may want to find out more
about. So we're going to add another couple of columns
to your inventory to explore your food/feelings patterns.

As you keep this diary, try not to judge your nonhunger
eating. Eating to get through a stressful period or to handle
a crisis is not necessarily bad. But that kind of eating
should be, as much as possible, a matter of choice. And
understanding more about specifically what feelings you're

having trouble with and when helps put the situation under your control.

DIARY #2
FOOD/FEELINGS

TIME	FOOD	HUNGER AMOUNT	FULLNESS LEVEL	LEVEL	MOOD	SITUATION

What Does Your Diary Say About Food and Feelings in Your Life?
Does the word angry appear often? Or bored or depressed? This is like a picture of your life. Look at it. Understand what you're dealing with.

Once you've done that, you can see if there are other options for coping. Maybe you can't fix your situation at once and eliminate those feelings, but maybe you can talk to a friend about them or begin to make the kinds of small changes we talked about in Chapter 12. If you decide you need to use food to cope with a feeling, that's okay. Making it a conscious choice puts it into your control, and that's a step in the right direction.

Also, don't neglect the effect of movement on your mood and on your impulse to eat. Moving is natural and healthy for human beings. Drinking Slim-Fast isn't.

SUGGESTIONS

1. Wait to start fixing dinner until you can feel your hunger. Use a low fat snack to tide you over while you fix it.

2. Think about the last time you were upset enough to eat in a way you wished you hadn't. Close your eyes and try to put yourself in that same mood. Now go turn on some very lively music, like a John Philip Sousa march, and march or dance around the room. Focus on your posture, your facial expression. Do this for at least five minutes. Do you feel any different?

3. The next time you are driving home thinking you're going to clean out the refrigerator when you get there, don't go into the house until you've walked briskly around the block for fifteen minutes. Too cold out? Climb up and down the stairs as long as you can. You may eat the food anyway. But you will feel more in control, and next time you may not. Or you may eat less. Small victories.

15
When Your Eating
Feels Compulsive

I used to try to eat normal breakfast, lunch, and dinner food. But what's normal?

WORKSHOP MEMBER

FOR SOME OF US, eating has become a matter of binges, starvation, and, perhaps, purges. We are capable, at moments, of eating more than your average fullback. At other times, we eat nothing at all. We have come to have a love/hate relationship with food. We are afraid of it and we feel controlled by it.

THE IDEAL FOOD DAY

If this is your situation, we'd like to present a method that can lead you to freedom. At the same time, it's a method that won't scare you with its lack of structure. It's designed to give you a genuine sense of control and a more realistic judgment about the power of food in your life.

To fear is one thing. To let fear grab you by the tail and swing you around is another.

KATHERINE PATERSON

What we suggest is that you plan an "ideal food" day. This is simply planning a day of eating that sounds good— that is, pleasurable—and giving it a try. The goal is to eat just what you planned to eat for one full day and feel satisfied by it.

The ideal food day is part of a learning process; it has nothing to do with dieting. You may have started dieting so early and so rigidly you have no recollection of your real food preferences. The ideal food day is an experiment that will help you get in touch with these preferences. It will also help you undo the damage that years of deprivation and guilty bingeing have done.

This is not a task at which you can fail. You can only learn. The process of creating weeks and months of ideal food days works because, while you are learning, you are creating situations in which you can experience control and success. Each satisfying experience adds to the confidence you need to try again tomorrow.

The ideal food day, unlike diet strategy, will not result in immediate weight loss. In all likelihood, it will allow your weight to stabilize near your current setpoint. It will give you time to make discoveries and slow changes without more of the yo-yo cycle. After you have made these discoveries, after you have experienced the feeling of meeting your body's needs and after you gain some sense of personal control, you have the option to make adjustments that will affect your setpoint in a positive way.

> *A cucumber should be well sliced, and dressed with pepper and vinegar, and then thrown out as good for nothing.*

> SAMUEL JOHNSON

For most people, the relief they experience when they give up dieting and take control over their own bodies more than compensates for the waiting period before they begin to lose weight. And consider the alternatives. Remember where the last three diets went when the deprivation ended. With this method, your weight may stay where it is for a while, but you won't have to start over again.

You begin by sitting down and writing out what food you think would make you happy for a full day. You don't plan a "reasonable diet" day or the other extreme, a binge. You won't need to binge if the experiment works. You will have a lot of these days to plan. Ideal day after ideal day. You don't have to cram all the forbidden goodies into twenty-four hours.

It may be difficult for you to identify things you really like to eat. If you have had the energy to keep a journal, look at the days you think you binged. Are your "binge foods" things you thoroughly enjoy? If so, think about incorporating them into your plan.

If even your binge foods are restricted to huge salads or saltines and jelly, try other ways of "remembering" what you love to eat. Is there something you see on other people's plates at restaurants that always makes you envious? What appeals to you, regardless of the fat or calories?

If you can remember a time before food became utterly restricted, search your memory for clues. When you went to the movies as a child, what did you get to eat at the concession stand? When you went out to eat with your family, what did you order? Did you used to *love* pork chops? Or baked potatoes?

Do your best to come up with foods that you genuinely enjoy. If you have real difficulty with this, try this journal for a week or two.

DIARY #3
FAVORED FOODS

TIME	FOOD	AMOUNT	WHAT WOULD HAVE MADE YOU HAPPY	AMOUNT

Cued by the foods that are serving as "stand-ins" for what you really want, you may be able to figure out some of the things you like to eat.

Now, plan a day in which you will eat only things you like, including some of these foods. Don't worry about nutrition. In the first place, a few days of no significant food value won't kill you. In the second place, what kind of nutrition are you getting now with starving and bingeing? Do you really think it could be worse?

As you plan, decide on amounts that also seem "reasonable" to you. It is not important that the package says three cookies equal one serving. You may need six or ten to satisfy you. Write it down. If the idea of going too far scares you, consider portion controls. There are lots of possibilities. You can buy things in small packages. You can put things in small packages yourself. You can even cook part of a cake mix. The thing to remember is that you're controlling the portions; they aren't controlling you. You can eat more than one package without guilt, but you will be aware of your eating.

After you've put down the foods you care about at the times you want to eat them, there will probably be blank spaces left in your day. Fill those in now. These are the places you don't have strong feelings or cravings. For example, the idea of juice and toast for breakfast might seem okay for some of you. (For others, it will be steak and eggs.)

Look carefully at your plan and make sure you've included enough to satisfy hunger and cravings for the whole day. And be sure you haven't copped out by writing angel food cake when you mean German chocolate cake.

Here are a couple of ideal food days. Marla's is very different from Kim's. Their bodies work differently, and they like different things. Together they should give you some idea of what we're talking about.

MARLA	KIM

Breakfast and morning

1 or 2 raisin bran muffins with jelly	2 cups leftover scalloped potatoes
2 packages of Lifesavers	2 or 3 cups of coffee
1 package of gum	1 slice of ham
2 Fannie Mac caramel lollipops	1 cup of applesauce
2 cups of coffee	6 to 10 Milky Way miniatures

Lunch and afternoon

Frozen yogurt sundae made with 1 ½ cups of frozen yogurt	Large serving of pasta with garlic and oil
1 whole cantaloupe	1 whole stalk of steamed broccoli
4 cookies	6 ounces of red wine
Reddi Wip light	2 or 3 ounces of pretzels
6 to 10 hard candies	8 ounces of orange juice
	2 or 3 caramel Nips

Dinner and evening

2 bialys with jelly	4 ounce steak
1 baked potato with bacon bits	1 baked potato with low-fat sour cream
2 or 3 pieces of fat-free pastry	1 whole sliced beefsteak tomato
A handful of crackers and jelly	2 slices of french bread and margarine
	6 ounces of red wine
	1 cup of chocolate frozen yogurt
	1 cup of coffee
	2 ounces of cognac

Neither of these two has planned what people might call a "normal" day of eating. But both of them were able to stick to what they planned to eat. At this stage, that is the important thing.

That's the second step. Follow your plan. Don't fudge by pulling back from what you've allotted yourself, by restricting yourself out of habit. Eat what you have planned to eat.

If you fall apart, meaning you don't stay with your food selection, notice what you ate instead. Maybe that's what you really wanted. Put those foods in tomorrow's plan and try again. Kim, for example, only came to the 6 to 10 Milky Way miniatures after having gone through Fig Newtons, sandwich cookies, and a smaller number of Milky Ways.

Just keep in mind that this is a process. You are going from one day to the next. You are slowly gathering information about your likes and experiencing the feeling that you do have some control.

THINGS TO TRY

1. Eat Hershey's Kisses for breakfast.
2. Shop when you're hungry.
3. Go to a country diner for dinner.
4. Drink a can of nondiet soda.
5. Eat an order of french fries for lunch.
6. Make yourself mashed potatoes and gravy for dinner.

Some days you will succeed. You will go through a whole day eating just what you planned to eat and feeling satisfied with it. You will gradually come to learn how to satisfy both physical and emotional needs. You will begin to eliminate the chaos in your eating and move toward making food a pleasure.

You are establishing eating patterns that you can begin

to use as a basis of change. When you don't know what you like to eat and want to eat and when, you can't work out a fat budget. You don't have a clue what your "expenses" are. But once you are out of the cycle of dieting and bingeing, you can begin the process we described in Chapter 8.

SUGGESTIONS

1. If you don't feel you need the whole ideal food day, planning can still help you. Make some simple plans about how to use your fat budget in advance. If you know you're going out to dinner, save up for it by having cereal and skim milk for breakfast. Then *thoroughly enjoy* your dinner.

2. Always have something around you really like just in case the urge hits you. This will help you avoid "grazing." If overdoing it worries you, try keeping this treat around in a way that takes a few minutes to prepare, a cake mix instead of a cake. This provides you "think time," and it's better than mindlessly finding your hand in an empty box.

3. Don't try to make up for a binge after it happens. If you binge in the afternoon, eat dinner anyway.

16
When It's a Matter of Life and Death

❧

Although the world is full of suffering, it is full also of the overcoming of it.

HELEN KELLER

NOW. THIS BOOK is, and is not, about eating disorders. It began with a look at the diet industry. For that reason alone, it would be insane to ignore eating disorders. They make up a significant part of the diet program business. More important, the diet industry plays a part in the *creation* of eating disorders. On a personal, individual level, it worsens the situations of its clients because of its emphasis on rigid dieting. On a larger level, it helps to foster a climate in which women develop unrealistic expectations and therefore make unreasonable demands on their bodies.

> *A recent South Carolina study of 13,000 schoolchildren reported that 15 percent had starved themselves or forced bulimic episodes in order to lose weight.*

If you suspect that your problems with food and weight go beyond those of the usual chronic dieter, or if you care about someone who may have more serious problems, read the following material carefully. We are going to describe the common eating disorders.[1]

And they are indeed *very* common. According to the National Association of Anorexia Nervosa and Associated Disorders, there are 8 million people in the United States who suffer from severe eating disorders such as anorexia and bulimia. About 7 million of them are girls and women.

If, after reading the profiles that follow, you feel your problem comes under this heading, do not under any circumstances consider going to a diet center. A diet could be deadly. Instead, call one of the people or organizations listed at the end of this chapter.

> *According to a University of Arizona study, 35 percent of all female athletes have some variety of pathological eating disorder.*

The following descriptions may not be complete or comprehensive, but they will give you an idea of what we're talking about when we say "eating disorder." You may recognize some of your own behaviors and wonder about yourself. Some of these characteristics are common among those who have simply been on and off diets all of their lives. Chronic dieters exhibit patterns of obsessions with food, fear of fat, and ritualized behavior. Without fear of seeming a hypochondriac, you need to evaluate how serious your problem is. If you have doubts, you should probably talk to a counselor.

ANOREXIA NERVOSA

If you are anorexic, you are probably a woman and probably young, but these are not absolutes. There is an increas-

---

1. The profiles in this chapter are based on the descriptions from the book *Surviving an Eating Disorder*, by Michele Siegel, Judith Brisman, and Margot Weinshel

ingly large number of male anorectics, and some women become anorectic later in life. You are intensely fearful of becoming obese, and this fear does not diminish when you lose weight. You have lost a considerable amount of weight that cannot be attributed to illness.

If you are anorectic, you are the only one who thinks you are fat. While others admire your slender figure—or are alarmed by your emaciated one—you fail to understand why they don't see the fat that you see when you look in the mirror.

You refuse to keep your weight within a normal range. You tell other people that you have "a very small frame" or "very fine bones" to justify your need for a below-average weight. You even believe that this is true.

You may very well have stopped menstruating.

You have extremely ritualized food behavior. We are not talking here about a need for hourly diet sodas. You may have limited your food choices to only three or four. When you eat a sandwich, you may cut it into bites and take as long as an hour to eat it.

If you have responsibility for the feeding of others, you pay a great deal of attention to food preparation for them, though you eat little or none of what is prepared.

BULIMIA

If you are bulimic, your eating gets out of control. You experience episodes of binge eating. Even while they are going on, you are aware of great discomfort and you know that the quantity you are eating is abnormal. After a binge, you attempt to purge yourself of the food. You may do this by vomiting. You may also do it by using laxatives or diuretics, by fasting or severely restricting your food intake for a period of time or even by intensive exercise. For example, you may follow a binge by walking or jogging for five or six hours. As your illness progresses, you may begin to purge yourself after smaller and smaller portions of food.

You are often depressed. You are also afraid that, once you start eating, you will be unable to stop.

Following a binge, you experience great self-loathing. You feel that you have been out of control, and this makes you lose respect for yourself.

COMPULSIVE EATING

You eat in many ways that make you feel ashamed. Sometimes, you binge. Other times you go on semi-starvation diets, which quickly fall apart.

You also engage in secret eating. You eat little in public but binge when you are alone. You hide food. You arrange your life so that you will not have to eat in front of others. Indeed, you restrict many of your activities because of shame over your weight and your eating habits.

You may have hypertension or experience fatigue that is related to your weight. You have, at times in your life, endured rapid and extreme weight gains.

Anorexia and bulimia have a higher death rate than any other mental illness, including clinical depression.

These profiles were not included just because there are people with eating disorders going to diet programs, where diet can be a matter of life and death. There is another reason. If you have been through the diet mill, if you are a "lifer," it is likely that you will find that some of the descriptions apply to you. Perhaps you will see yourself in a sentence from one list and a sentence from another. Or, maybe you will think the symptoms sound familiar but question whether your behavior is that extreme.

We want you to think about that. There is a fine line between chronic dieting and a subclinical eating disorder (one not exhibiting all the symptoms). It is our feeling and the opinion of many experts that diet programs, by fostering the diet mentality, encourage disordered eating. This may not occur while the person is in the program but show up as rebound behavior. As a result, the individual may go back to that or another program out of fear, seeking the structure and accountability that she hopes will keep her under control.

Some clients reported that, after being on diet programs, their own behavior worsened into full-blown bulimia or compulsive eating. This is not surprising. For one thing, a diet program is focused on food and weight but rarely addresses more than the symptom. Second, in most programs, counselors are not equipped by education or background to do more than deal with surface issues. Finally, you may not even be ready to tackle food behaviors until you deal with other issues in your life. If you are in a diet program, even if your eating behavior does not get worse, you will continue to believe you can control your life by controlling food. You will never get beyond that to your real problems.

In the foreword to *Overcoming Overeating,* Janet Polivy, an eating disorder therapist, states: "Clinicians such as Hirschmann and Munter have simultaneously reached the same conclusion [as other therapists) on the basis of their exposure to eating-disordered clients. The 'compulsive eating' that plagues their clients is eating out of sync with the body's natural needs; it is eating for all the wrong reasons. And how does such compulsive overeating ... arise? Almost invariably, it is the result of dieting."

Dieting is defined very simply. It involves learning to give preference to "the diet allowance" over the body's demands. The more extreme and rigid the diet, the less in touch people are with their physical needs and the less they trust their own bodies. This is particularly true because, at some point, this perversity breaks down and the opposite behavior—gluttony—takes over. And still, the body is not acknowledged; neither deprivation nor gluttony meets the body's needs.

Eventually if the deprivation is intense enough, food comes to fill every sort of emotional and physical emptiness, because it wasn't available when needed. The logical end of this process is disordered eating on a regular basis, disordered body image, and an all-consuming focusing on food and weight.

If you feel that your eating has elements of this kind of disorder, we suggest that you get professional help. Use the information in Chapter 13 to guide you.

Inevitably, the question of hospitalization comes up in extreme cases of anorexia or morbid obesity combined with complications that can be immediately life threatening. The issue also arises because many hospitals now offer short-term eating disorder programs involving six weeks of hospitalization. The stay includes monitored eating, individual counseling, group therapy, education on nutrition, and often encouragement of such healthful outlets as exercise sessions, art therapy, and so forth. Is this for you?

There may have been a time when this was a good choice, and there may still be programs that offer excellent staff and services. The impact of the insurance industry, however, has been to lessen the quality and benefit of hospitalization as a solution. In discussing these programs with social workers (one of whom is employed by an insurance company to evaluate hospitalization), we found that the feeling was generally negative. Only those who were not familiar with the long-term efforts required to deal with eating disorders felt these programs had merit. At a recent conference, a psychologist and author of one of these hospital programs for bulimics admitted that this six-week program was just a start to ongoing treatment.

There are some therapists who feel that the hospital can give the patient a respite from the immediate situation contributing to the eating disorder, that in a hospital setting there is a chance for intense focus and guidance. But the majority of professionals feel that hospitalization is a last resort. If it is required for medical intervention, there is no choice. We have interviewed several compulsive eaters who went through six-week programs for morbid obesity. They lost many pounds (more than fifty in each case), were exposed to intense, daily behavior modification drills, and still gained the weight back after hospitalization.

As we have been saying in every other chapter in this book, altering chronic unhealthy eating patterns takes time. It must be approached slowly and with awareness of all other areas of the individual's life.

17
A Note for Men

⌐━⌐

My doctor says I'm a heart attack waiting to happen. I can't go back there until I drop at least thirty pounds.

DIET PROGRAM CLIENT

FOR MEN, THE weight crunch usually comes in their thirties or later. Up to that time, one of two things has been true. Either you've gotten by with a little extra weight because, frankly, men can. Or you've been active enough that it hasn't been a problem.

There's no denying that men "get by" with a lot more in the realm of weight than women do. In the first place, your higher percentage of lean body mass means that you do not gain weight as easily as a woman. Every time you move, you burn more calories than a similarly healthy woman. And then, like it or not, our society places more value on what a man *does* and on how a woman *looks*. A man who is a successful attorney, with all the trappings to accompany that position, doesn't even have to think about an extra ten pounds. If he's a perfectionist, he may, but he doesn't really have to.

Even while growing up, boys have a much larger margin for error. Being "huskier" than other kids can be an advantage. You aren't fat; you're good material for the football team.

Of course, this is a generalization. And even if you have managed to "get by," there may have been pain and unhappiness along the way. Not every chubby boy is a potential fullback. Your story may sound more like this.

"In school I was known as Fat Phil. It was painful. I developed an image of myself as unacceptable, especially to the girls around me. When I look back, I really wasn't terribly fat, just huskier than other kids. You know the ones—long, lanky, and undeveloped. But it became an issue.

"I never went on a formal diet. I just struggled with ideas of my own occasionally, then gave up. It became more serious five years ago, when I gave up smoking. At the same time I was going through a very depressing period, a dragged-out divorce. My weight jumped another twenty pounds. The doctor is on my back. I feel like I need help, but I don't know where to go. I can't see walking into a lobby full of women at Jenny Craig. That's why I came to this workshop."

Even in Phil's case, the problem didn't get his full attention until he began to slow down. You may have had the same experience. Your situation may be something like this. Until now, you didn't have to do much more than take out the garbage and mow the lawn in order to keep your weight under control. But now you have a riding mower, and your teenager wrestles the garbage cans. Then, too, you used to stay home on the weekends and play with the kids—build them a swing set, teach them to catch and hit, take them on bike rides. Now they're out on their own and you're close enough to vice president that you bring work home with you. You have a PC in the spare room and, when you're finished with the sales projections, you find yourself exploring new software.

> *After thirty, a body has a mind of its own.*
>
> BETTE MIDLER

Your weight has begun to increase with inactivity. And there's a good chance that you didn't begin to worry about it until your doctor turned to you and said, "Blood pressure's getting a little high." Then you began to worry a lot.

"If I want good medical insurance," says Jay, "I have to drop fifty pounds."

"I do not want to hear what the doctor has to say until I've lost twenty pounds. His lectures only depress me. I am more likely to cheer myself up with food."

Now, we won't go on at any length about doctors who push weight loss instead of exercise and good nutrition as a goal, and we won't say what we think of doctors who put numbers on the weight loss. Suffice it to say that a lot of men have been thrown into a muck sweat by doctors who don't seem to have a clue that what they're doing is destructive.

If your doctor says to lose weight, ask questions. What is the specific medical problem he or she is concerned about? What research is there to indicate that it is affected by weight? Show your doctor pages 106–110 of this book and talk about the findings we report there. Ask if what's really at issue isn't becoming fit by gradually lowering the fat in your diet and getting more exercise. Then start doing it.

GETTING STARTED

You have some real advantages in this business. Your body is Bailey's "better butter burner" biologically. And you're less likely than a woman to have spent years dieting, so you may not have messed up your metabolism and screwed up your setpoint.

Now for your disadvantages. You may not have a clue about nutrition. And you probably don't control what goes into your mouth. There may very well be a woman in your life who picks out, prepares, and serves you your food. "My wife does all the cooking," says Webster. "I eat whatever is in the house, if it's cookies for the kids or three helpings of dinner. When I'm tired, looking for relaxation, diversion, I eat whatever's around.'' And whatever's around is what your wife picked up at the store. In addition, if your doctor has warned you about your weight, your wife or girlfriend may now be acting as a policeman, enforcing anti-hamburger statutes.

> Among the most disheartening and dangerous of . . . advisors, you will often find those closest to you, your dearest friends, members of your own family, perhaps, loving, anxious, and knowing nothing whatever.
>
> MINNIE MADDERN FISKE

Well, when Claire Huxtable, on ''The Cosby Show,'' treats Cliff like a child, scolding him for his never-ending attempts to indulge in ''bacon burger *dawgs*,'' it's not only insulting to men, it's very bad weight control practice. Most men already have inclinations toward independent action. Aren't you the guys who won't stop at a gas station for directions and hate to call a plumber? That independence can be your biggest advantage in this business of weight.

For one thing, it's probably kept you away from the diet centers, that and the disinclination to enter a ''woman's world.'' If you've been to a diet program, the chances are very good that you enrolled in a medically supervised fast such as Optifast or that you joined a support group such as TOPS. You may have joined Weight Watchers somewhere along the line. The few of you who show up at Nutri/System and Jenny Craig follow the same quick-loss-quick-regain pattern that women do. If you've done it more than once, you've probably suffered the same loss of self-esteem.

But most of you don't ask anyone else for help, with the possible exception of your wife.

Since being in charge of your own program is such an important part of a successful approach to weight control, this can be, as we said, a good thing. But it needs to be accompanied by some knowledge of what you're doing. We interviewed, in a restaurant, a couple who were both concerned about their weight. The husband indicated his impatience with his wife's lack of self-control when she ordered a barbecued beef sandwich, and then he ordered a Caesar salad. Depending on the recipes used, it was a toss-up which one was getting more fat. She may even have had the edge.

Another man recently asked us, "Does olive oil have fat in it?"

Now, while the women reading this chapter fall off their chairs laughing, we will explain to some of you men that oil *is* fat. And just so you won't think we're too impressed with our superior knowledge, we'll admit that there was a time when we thought an *oil change* involved switching brands.

In the beginning years of the women's movement, thousands of women went out and took auto repair classes as a way of gaining control over their lives. Now, maybe it's time for thousands of men to sign up for nutrition classes for the same reason. They're offered at most YMCAs and YWCAs and at lots of community colleges. (If you can't find one in your area, there are books. We've included a couple of good ones in the Appendix.) Otherwise, you're going to have to put up with the same kind of condescending bull from women about food that women used to put up with from men about cars.

LOOKING AT YOUR EATING PATTERNS

So you're in control and you're learning about nutrition. Now, as we stressed in earlier chapters, you need to take a look at what you eat and when. If a formal record of your eating is out of the question, compromise. At the end of one or two typical days, make a list of the things you ate. This cannot take more than five minutes.

Here are the simple changes that one man made with a food journal and a nutrition guide, using the guidelines in Chapter 10.

ANDREW'S JOURNAL

TIME	FOOD	CALORIES	FAT GRAMS
7:30	jelly-filled Dunkin' Donuts	220	9
	1 cup of coffee with 2 tablespoons cream	80	6
3:00	Greek salad with 2 ounces of feta cheese and 3 tablespoons of dressing	400	42
	5 Lifesavers	50	0
	1 package of gum	50	0
5:00	2 light beers	192	10
	1 small bag of potato chips	200	15
7:00	2 pieces of bbq chicken (2 whole chicken breasts)	706	28
	baked potato with 1 teaspoon butter	205	4
	1 slice vienna bread with 1 teaspoon butter	125	4
9:30	2 chocolate brownies	320	14
	handful of peanuts (½ ounce)	75	7
	TOTAL	2623	fat grams x 9 = 1251

All right. Andrew takes in 2,623 calories total and 1,251 of those calories come from fat. In other words, 48 percent of Andrew's caloric intake (1251 divided by 2623) is from fat. If Andrew wants to change his setpoint, he needs to reduce that percentage. The question is whether he can do it without making himself feel deprived.

This is how Andrew decided he could restructure the day.

ANDREW'S REVISED JOURNAL

TIME	FOOD	CALORIES	FAT	FAT SAVED
7:30	*jelly-filled Dunkin' Donuts*	220	9	0
	1 cup of coffee with 2 tablespoons milk	60	4	2
3:00	*Greek salad with 1 ounce of feta cheese and 1 ½ tablespoons of dressing*	280	22	20
	chunk of bread	100	0	
	5 Lifesavers	50	0	
	1 package of gum	50	0	
5:00	*1 regular beer*	147	5	5
	1 small bag of pretzels	165	1.5	13.5
7:00	*2 pieces of bbq chicken (2 whole chicken breasts without the skin)*	584	9	19
	baked potato with 2 tablespoons of non-fat sour cream instead of butter	230	0	4
	1 slice vienna bread with 1 teaspoon lowfat margarine instead of butter	110	2	2

TIME	FOOD	CALORIES	FAT	FAT SAVED
9:30	2 chocolate brownies	320	14	0
	skipped peanuts	0	0	75
	TOTAL	2316	66.5	72.5
			fat grams x	9
				= 599

Andrew has cut his fat percentage more than in half without making radical changes in type of food or amount. The changes may not be ones you could live with, but they were ones he could live with.

For example, Andrew doesn't really care about the difference between cream and milk in his coffee. It's not a big deal to him. As for the changes in his Greek salad lunch, he actually *prefers* to have bread with his meal and less dressing. It just never occurred to him to order the dressing on the side, and he thought bread was fattening. Cutting down to one beer after work sounded just fine, especially when he realized that he didn't have to drink light. And pretzels were an acceptable substitute for potato chips because he really only wanted something salty to go with his beer.

A point here about alcohol. Beer, wine, and liquor don't actually have fat in them. However, your body metabolizes alcohol in the same way as fat. Nutritionists therefore usually count one drink (six ounces of wine, twelve ounces of beer, or one and a half ounces of hard liquor) as five fat grams. The reason Andrew can have regular beer is that most brewers now lower the calories in beer by reducing the carbohydrates, not the alcohol. In terms of fat content, a light beer isn't any better than a regular beer, *unless* it has a lower alcohol content. So why skimp on taste?

Chicken skin was also not something Andrew cared about preserving, and it wasn't that much trouble to remove it. In fact, Andrew didn't even bother buying skinless chicken breasts at a dollar a pound more.

And as for the way he fixed his potato, Andrew had given up sour cream, which he preferred, years ago, because it was fattening. Butter was nowhere near as satisfying to him, but he didn't like dry potatoes. When Andrew tried one of the new fat-free sour cream substitutes, he was thrilled to have the old sour cream taste back and he gave up the butter without a qualm. Andrew kept the dessert he really loved and gave up the peanuts he ate just because they were there.

Andrew has not gone on another diet. Nothing he gave up is something he cares about. He still has his jelly doughnut in the morning and his beer after work. He has almost the same lunch he had before and almost the same dinner.

He also made these changes slowly. He got used to one of them before he went on to another. And that is critical. If you decide to take the bull by the horns and just slash the fat in your diet overnight, two things are likely to happen. First, your metabolism will suffer as it would from any other drastic calorie reduction. Second, you're very unlikely to stick with your changes.

Andrew had help making his changes because he consulted an individual weight control counselor who knew a lot about what kinds of low-fat foods are available. If you're going to try this on your own, you also need to know what's available today on the supermarket shelves.

So, is there any reason you can't go shopping?

Shopping?

Oh, don't be such a baby. You can survive a trip or two to the mall. Even if you don't plan to shop regularly, give yourself a break. There's a whole new world out there you may not know about, especially if no one else in the house is diet-conscious. Take a stroll down the aisles of your grocery store and make yourself familiar with all the healthy low-fat alternatives. Then you can at least add your choices to your wife's grocery list.

GETTING A MOVE ON

Now we come to the second and perhaps more important of the two fronts on which you need to attack this problem.

You probably got where you are by reducing your level of physical activity. And you can get out of it by increasing said level.

Take Frank, for example. After his wife died, he spent several very lonely years. One of the reasons he hesitated asking a woman out is that he was five six and a little on the chubby side. At forty-five, having spent twenty-five years behind a desk, he had a fairly good-sized paunch and was sure he needed to lose twenty pounds.

Frank and his wife had dieted regularly together over the years. They joined Weight Watchers, took trips to a "fat farm," lived on Metrecal (the early version of liquid diets). He lost the weight pretty easily, gained it even more easily.

Now, however, Frank was starting over on his own. With a counselor, he decided the first thing affecting him was the fact that he didn't cook. Most of his meals were carry-out or junk. So he started cooking and it gave him a wonderful sense of control over his life. He didn't toss all his treats in the trash, as he once would have. He settled, instead, for one or two beers instead of three or four. He found he could be happy with chicken, pasta, or rice and beans for a lot of his meals. As long as he could still have a hamburger once during the week, he was fine. He still had desserts and enjoyed bread and potatoes. He felt much healthier.

> *Excess on occasion is exhilarating. It prevents moderation from acquiring the deadening effect of a habit.*
>
> W. SOMERSET MAUGHAM

But he wasn't really losing a lot of weight.

That's when he decided to look at the reality of his situation. At forty-five, he had a lifelong history of yo-yo dieting. His setpoint had been seriously affected by this history. *The chances he could once more weigh what he had at twenty-five were not good.*

That was Frank's reality, and it led to his dealing with his situation in a way that made sense to him.

He decided he might never be twenty pounds lighter, but he could be fitter. He could join a health club (not a bad idea for meeting people either) and make the extra pounds look a lot better.

The health club was the change Frank needed. He did aerobics and weights four times a week. He decided to work with the club trainer, who was a real motivator. As Frank gradually changed fat to muscle, he looked different but he didn't see a big drop in pounds. He was happy enough with his appearance that he didn't get discouraged by the scale. A year later Frank is still working out, is eating the same way, and is down about ten pounds. He doesn't really feel the need to lose any more.

Frank's approach is right for him, but that doesn't mean it would be right for you. Part of your reality might be that you never have and never will join an aerobics class. Or that you don't have the time or money for a health club. If that's the case, you need to be creative.

Check out every possibility for physical activity in your area. Call up the YMCA, the park district, a community center. See what they have that fits your schedule. Look in the entertainment section of your local newspaper. If you live anywhere but in a very small town, you'll be surprised at all the things going on. You should find lists of biking, hiking, and walking clubs. City recreational classes will be listed.

Look for activities offered for the family, things you can do with your children. This gives you additional motivation, especially if your busy schedule has limited the time you spend with the family. We know of parents who take skating or swimming classes with children or play family volleyball.

Put up a basketball hoop on your garage. Then, next time you're having friends over for dinner, tell them to wear their grungies and be prepared to shoot some hoops before the barbecue. This has the added advantage of cutting down on beer consumption and boring conversations.

Encourage outings for your family that are primarily

walking. Go to the woods, the shoreline (if you are lucky enough to live near one), the zoo, or the city's botanical gardens.

For other help, Covert Bailey's *Fit or Fat* is ideal reading for men.

One final suggestion. Have a body-fat test. Many community centers do them with calipers, for a nominal fee. Your percentage of body fat is a lot more meaningful than your poundage. This is particularly true of "big men." If your weight has never matched the Metropolitan Life height/weight chart, but your body fat is 20 percent or less, don't give your weight another thought.

You're fine.

And now, here's that other set of rules we promised you, from the immortal Satchel Paige.

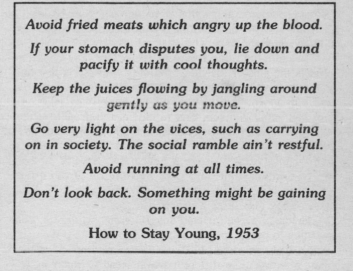

Avoid fried meats which angry up the blood.

If your stomach disputes you, lie down and pacify it with cool thoughts.

Keep the juices flowing by jangling around gently as you move.

Go very light on the vices, such as carrying on in society. The social ramble ain't restful.

Avoid running at all times.

Don't look back. Something might be gaining on you.

How to Stay Young, 1953

Appendix: Resources

WE SUGGESTED EARLIER that you toss out your scale. It's probably a good idea to donate your diet books to the next church rummage sale.

What falls into this category? Basically, any book that repeats the sins of the diet programs. Any book that tells you exactly what to eat and what not to eat, when to eat, and how to eat. And definitely any book that makes you feel bad about yourself, that diminishes your self-esteem.

If you haven't read anything but diet books until now, we'd like to recommend some books that can be very helpful in starting you on a new track. Several of them we've mentioned already. Like *Feeding on Dreams*, they offer research and observations showing why diets don't work. They also offer alternative ideas.

The books we've selected cover a variety of topics, from nutrition to psychology to behavior modification. We don't expect that each one will have the same impact on you. They affected us in different ways. Read as many as you can. If you are not a reader by nature, just thumb through or look at the introduction.

In this book, we have stressed that there are many elements to almost any person's struggle with weight. Most of these books deal with only one element. It's going to be up to you to see the issues they discuss as only one part of the whole picture.

Start with a book that addresses your biggest obstacle. If the book seems to ring true for you, resist the notion to make your life and your problems fit the pattern the book presents. Use what makes sense, or at least think about what makes sense, and then move on. If you are already very familiar with certain issues, such as the benefits of exercise or the feminist perspective on body image, start with the other recommendations.

It is our feeling that the following authors are the best in their field and are worthy of your attention.

THE BIG GUYS

Covert Bailey, *The New Fit or Fat* (Boston: Houghton Mifflin, 1991)

Few books or authors have had such a positive impact on chronic dieters as Bailey's *Fit or Fat*. There are many people whose lives were changed when the first book came out more than fifteen years ago. It was the first clear consumer-oriented explanation of why low-calorie dieting is ineffective and counterproductive in weight control.

By the time his second book, *The New Fit or Fat,* was published in 1991, Bailey's writing had made exercise converts of thousands of former dieters. In the new edition, he starts by saying, in effect, ''I told you not to diet in my first book and I'm still telling you not to diet.'' The new book sums up some of the key points that were presented in the first book but adds to the reader's understanding by including the most current research in diet and exercise physiology.

For instance, in *The New Fit or Fat,* Bailey explains why it is no longer necessary to be a slave to pulse taking. He explains how to identify and use ''perceived exertion level.'' He also clarifies the fitness/fatness relationship. He explains at much greater length than we were able to in this book *why* a fat body stores fat and a lean body is a ''better butter burner.'' There are also chapters on how to get an exercise start and on the most frequently asked questions on diet and exercise.

Bailey's writing is easy to understand and very funny. This helps a lot if you have resisted exercise in favor of food deprivation. When you finish reading Bailey's book, it is almost impossible not to feel real motivation. You want to grab your walking shoes and give it a try.

Covert Bailey and Lea Bishop: *The Fit or Fat Woman* (Boston: Houghton Mifflin, 1989)

You may want to read *The New Fit or Fat* before you read about unique concerns for women. Although the author does summarize his antidiet/pro-exercise arguments in this book, there is more on the fitness/fatness theory in the first book.

The Fit or Fat Woman is very useful in guiding a woman reader to set more realistic exercise goals. The authors discuss at length the natural predisposition for women to carry a higher percentage of body fat than men and how this affects their weight. The book also includes chapters on depression, PMS, anorexia, and bulimia. There is something very refreshing in hearing a man address the issue of weight as a social and cultural issue in today's world.

If you have wasted time trying to meet unrealistic goals of thinness and "fitness," *The Fit or Fat Woman* will give you new options and change your perspective. Besides, there's a chapter called "Healthy Women Do Jiggle!"

William Bennett and Joel Gurin, *The Dieter's Dilemma* (New York: Basic Books, 1982)

Curious as to how your body really works? This might be the first book to try. You will probably have to get it from the library or order it from your bookstore. You may not find it as entertaining as Bailey's *Fit or Fat,* but it is a more comprehensive presentation of human physiology. The authors present impressive research to support their antidiet stand. If the studies get a little slow or tedious, go to the areas of personal interest.

The best reason for suggesting this book is that it completcly explodes all the accepted diet myths. After a dozen or so studies, you can put aside any thought that instability, lack of discipline, or deep-seated neurotic feelings are the primary causes of fat bodies.

Jane R. Hirschmann and Carol H. Munter, *Overcoming Overeating* (New York: Ballantine Books, 1989)

If you think of yourself as a compulsive eater, trapped in an addictive cycle of food and diets, this book will probably open your mind to new thinking. It will certainly put your food problems in a healthier and more constructive light. Hirschmann and Munter use every conceivable approach to help you see that compulsive eating is not crazy but is the flip side of deprivation.

Their concepts are exciting and innovative. *Overcoming Overeating* focuses on dumping diets, realizing the negative impact of self-deprivation, and learning to eat when and what you want. The goal, or the end of this process, is getting to a place called feeding on demand.

Not everyone can go the whole nine yards. We have mentioned a number of times in this book that you need to start where you are now. Do the best you can, while still maintaining a level of emotional comfort. Your job is to learn about your own hunger, acknowledge it, and feed it appropriately. Dieting is a difficult pattern to undo; you will need to have a lot of patience with yourself. Read this book with the idea that this is the direction you want to travel.

Susie Orbach, *Fat Is a Feminist Issue II* (New York: Berkeley Books, 1982)

The original book by Susie Orbach, *Fat Is a Feminist Issue* (published in 1978), is now considered a classic in feminist literature. It is also a landmark work in the study of cultural influences on women and their bodies. The first book is largely a social and historical analysis of how women came to feel as they do about their bodies and food.

When you read *Fat Is a Feminist Issue*, you have a chance to question the clichés about eating as neurosis, fat and character, and self-destructive behavior and begin to view food behavior as positive and a part of survival. In a world where women do not have much of a voice, Orbach says, your body becomes a form of self-expression; it speaks for you.

Orbach has some excellent thoughts on the benefits of support groups, along with her own experiences in working with such a group.

In *Fat Is a Feminist Issue II,* you will find a couple of chapters that go over the important ideas in the first book. This second book, however, goes beyond theory, beyond social and political analysis, to techniques for discovering the "meaning" of your eating patterns. It includes fantasy exercises, followed by "consciousness-raising" questions that, used in a group or alone, are splendid tools for finding your own answers to questions that influence your weight more than a chocolate éclair.

Geneen Roth, *Feeding the Hungry Heart* (New York: Signet Books, 1983)
Geneen Roth, *Breaking Free from Compulsive Eating* (New York: Signet Books, 1984)

These two Roth books have been paired because, in some sense, they go together, although you may decide to read only one of them.

Feeding the Hungry Heart is an insightful and compassionate look into the world of people who have suffered greatly from their relationship to food. If you have felt isolated from everyone and everything in the world around you because of your problems with food, this book can be tremendously important in helping you see you are not alone, you are not strange, and you are not at fault. The book has a powerful emotional impact on readers, maybe more than you are ready for. If you find yourself greatly upset by the book, you might want to read it only as part of your work with a support group or a counselor.

The other consideration, when reading this book, is that you may identify so much with the author's experiences that you lose your own experience. You might forget the reality of the years of physical deprivation that contributed to your present situation and fall into thinking that your problems with food are entirely the result of deep and unresolved emotional conflict. Even if you have emotional issues to work on—some that are the result of dieting and others that have nothing to do with your relationship with food—keep in mind that resolving these issues is *only part of the picture.*

Breaking Free from Compulsive Eating was Roth's second book. This book attempts to pick up where *Feeding the Hungry Heart* ends. It is more of a "how to" book, which was inspired by reader response to the first book. The audience, finding themselves in the original stories, also discovered they did not know what to do with the insights. Roth's second book is about how to assess where you are and then walk away from deprivational dieting. *Breaking Free from Compulsive Eating* incorporates the views of other feminist authors, namely that food and weight are not matters of moral judgment and that both serve to help you survive.

The book also covers some of the points usually stressed by behavioral therapists. Again we caution you to use only what makes sense to you. There are suggestions, similar to those in this book, to help you get in touch with physical needs for food. There are suggestions to help you recognize and work around nonhunger eating. If you think it might help, give it a chance.

The focus of Roth's book is relearning self-trust, identifying hunger and other needs, and discovering better ways to meet these needs. It seems to connect with many readers because she writes honestly about her own experiences and those of people in her workshop. The book is very gentle and humane.

Melpomene Institute, *The Bodywise Woman* (New York: Prentice Hall Press, 1990)

This book, along with a number of other publications from the Melpomene Institute for Women's Health Research, is a real jewel. Unfortunately, it is not one you are likely to find except in a women's bookstore or in the library. It's worth the effort to find it or to order it. The book is filled with information and exercises on body image and self-acceptance. Much of it is consciousness-raising, giving you the opportunity and encouragement to figure out what is realistic and best for you.

The suggestions in *The Bodywise Woman* are down-to-earth and doable. We were especially impressed with the body-image section of the book and with suggested approaches to getting started on an exercise program. Most important, the emphasis is on an active healthy lifestyle, not on a diet.

If you are unable to find this book, you can order a packet of body-image materials directly from the Melpomene Institute for $10. Look under **Organizations** in this Appendix for the address.

Judith Rodin, *Body Traps* (New York: William Morrow, 1992)

Judith Rodin takes an "out-of-body" approach to the question of body images. That is, she tackles the various obsessions in our lives that make us exaggerate the importance of body size and shape. The easy-to-read book deals with the vanity trap, the shame trap, the competition trap, and even the fitness trap, offering real insight based on solid research. The book is sprinkled with consciousness-raising inventories and questionnaires that are very useful in helping the reader think about values and priorities in these various areas. It also contains exercises for dealing with and minimizing the destructiveness of the various life "traps."

The tone of this book is particularly appealing. It is sensible and sensitive, never falling into emotionalism, even while it deals with some strongly emotional issues. It is also one of the few books in this area that is genuinely nonspecific with regard to gender while strongly acknowledging feminist principles.

Karen J. Bellerson, *The Complete & Up-to-Date Fat Book* (Garden City Park, New York: Avery Publishing Group, 1993)

You need at least one source of accurate, complete information on the fat in your present diet. This is one of several good books around. We recommend this paperback here because it lists fat grams and percentage of calories from fat and includes generic listings, brand names, and popular fast-food items. Every listing has a portion size, and this is very important. Most of us look at the label, see three fat grams, and look no further. But if the can holds three portions, then eating the whole thing, which may be what you want to do, gives you nine grams of fat, a considerable difference.

OTHER BOOKS WITH GOOD IDEAS

James Ferguson, *Habits Not Diets* (Palo Alto: Bull Publishing, 1988)

If you like structure, workbooks, and making notes, *Habits Not Diets* will be very useful in organizing your thinking. This book is *strictly* behaviorist. There is not a lot of theory or explanation, but there are pages of charts, questions, and graphs to help to identify, record, and change behavior.

Use this book as an additional aid, very slowly and carefully. Don't try to go through the dozens of changes quickly. Remember, "only if it helps." Otherwise, you will have a behavioral *diet*.

Adelle Davis, *Let's Eat Right to Keep Fit* (New York: NAL-Dutton, 1970)

Are you really motivated to improve your health in addition to dealing with your weight? If you don't have much of a background in nutrition, you probably should get yourself one complete source. Although Davis's book has been around for a long time it has actually gained respect and credibility over the years. She was well ahead of her time in suggesting that proper nutrition was a form of disease prevention. Her book describes all the nutrients, their impact on your body, and the best food sources for each of the vitamins and minerals. It contains all the basics you need to make more informed food choices.

Bernard Gutin and Gail Kessler, *The High Energy Factor* (New York: Random House, 1982)

This book covers much of the information in *Fit or Fat* and *The Dieter's Dilemma,* but it adds some explanations of how your body works that do not appear in the other two books. Read it if you find you are still considering another diet instead of the fitness approach. What makes *The High Energy Factor* unique is that it looks very closely at movement per se, at changing to an active life-style rather than exercise isolated from life. It includes a great deal of information on the various types of exercise and how they add to the total fitness picture.

Marilyn Lawrence, *Fed Up and Hungry: Woman, Oppression, and Food* (New York: Peter Bedrick Books, 1987)

This anthology is the best professional "sampling" of anti-diet ideas. It contains fifteen articles by therapists who specialize in different aspects of eating disorders. *Fed Up and Hungry* is the kind of book that produces almost ongoing "aha" experiences. No matter how much you think you already know about yourself, your food behavior and how to "fix" things, all of the authors are provocative and open your eyes to fresh visions and ideas.

Among the best chapters are "Boundaries: One Way Mirror to the Self" by Mira Dana; "Women's Anger and Compulsive Eating," by Bunny Epstein; and "Self-Help Groups: The Agony and the Ecstasy," by Katina Noble. If your reading time is limited, *Fed Up and Hungry* is a wonderful selection of ideas.

Nancy Roberts, *Breaking All the Rules* (New York: Signet, 1983)

We hope that somewhere while reading *Feeding on Dreams* you found yourself feeling strong and sound about your body, that you felt like saying "This is me, damn it, and the world is going to meet me on my terms." If you did, don't miss the treat of indulging in Nancy Roberts's book. She writes with insight, compassion, and humor about having the world meet you halfway. She covers every aspect of life as a larger woman in an unforgiving world (you have to do the forgiving). She tells her own story and what made her decide to opt for self-acceptance rather than a life of diets. The book has wonderful practical tips on makeup, clothing (even sewing), and exercise. Give yourself a break and read it.

Geneen Roth, When Food Is Love (New York: Signet, 1992)

When Food Is Love is in many ways like Geneen Roth's first book, Feeding the Hungry Heart. It is autobiographical and gives the same feeling of intimacy and connection. We include this book here because Ms. Roth is very plain in describing the extent of her own success and "failure" to come to terms with food and her body. When Food Is Love conveys the sense of journey (not cure) very clearly. Roth is writing about another stage in the process of self-discovery. It is very important, no matter what place you are in, to realize that this is a growth process. It does not have a well-defined end, like losing thirty pounds before summer. The road we all travel is strewn with ruts and wrong turns.

All of Geneen Roth's books seem to have a high identification quotient, especially for people who have suffered greatly from their relationship with food, or for anyone who has been waging a battle with food for a very long time.

BOOKS FOR SPECIAL INTERESTS

Ellen Bass and Laura Davis, The Courage to Heal: A Guide for Women Survivors of Child Sexual Abuse (New York: Harper and Row, 1988)

This book is included because the problems of many women with food (and body image) have at least part of their origin in sexual abuse. If you only suspect you are an incest survivor, this book will help you to validate and understand childhood experiences. If you are already aware of sexual abuse or incest in your past, this book can be a powerful *adjunct* to individual counseling or group support. We want to make it clear that incest survivors need more than a book can provide to resolve very difficult issues.

Joan Jacobs Brumberg, *Fasting Girls: The Emergence of Anorexia Nervosa as a Modern Disease* (New York: Penguin Books, 1988)

Fasting Girls is a powerful, intellectual look at the history, etiology, and modern manifestations of eating disorders, particularly anorexia. It's absolutely fascinating. It will provide information, validation, and understanding but it is *definitely not* a substitute for counseling.

Kim Chernin, *The Obsession: Reflections on the Tyranny of Slenderness* (New York: Harper Colophon Books, 1981)

Kim Chernin, *The Hungry Self: Women, Eating and Identity* (New York: Times Books, 1985)

These two books will be of interest if you are a woman who is curious about the origins of your own eating disorders. Like Susie Orbach and Joan Brumberg, the author links cultural and social change with the development of food fetishes, diets, and body-image obsession. Chernin is a highly respected therapist and author on the subject of eating disorders. *The Hungry Self* is unique in seeing the key to disordered eating in the dynamics of mother-daughter relationships.

Edward Remington, Garth Fisher, and Edward Parent, *How to Lower Your Fat Thermostat* (Provo: Vitality House, 1983)

Edward Remington, Garth Fisher, and Edward Parent, *How to Lower Your Fat Thermostat Recipes* (Provo: Vitality House, 1984)

Do you really want to know what happens to dietary fat in your body? Are you curious about the journey of french fries from your mouth to your hips? The first book contains a lot of valuable nutritional information about the metabolism of fat and refined carbohydrates. To the credit of the authors they state that the whole issue of behavior modification and overweight needs to be reevaluated and updated. They further state that psychological problems, if significant, require professional intervention and that they are beyond the scope of their book. Good for them.

The second book is one of the best low-fat cookbooks on the market. It is especially helpful if used in conjunction with the theory of *How to Lower Your Fat Thermostat*. The book is attractively presented, easy to follow, and filled with nutritional information. Most of the recipes are simple, requiring only a few ingredients and no more than three or four steps. Every recipe comes with a nutritional analysis that includes fat grams (and percentage of fat), sodium, and cholesterol along with calories per portion.

Michele Siegel, Judith Brisman, and Margot Weinshel, *Surviving an Eating Disorder* (New York: Harper and Row, 1988)

If you are the parent, friend, or mate of someone who appears to be suffering with weight and food problems, you are probably unsure of the kind of help they need and may be aware that your intervention has been making things worse. *Surviving an Eating Disorder* will answer many of your questions. It suggests ways you can be supportive, encourage the individual to get help, and so forth. Most important, the book suggests when and how to find professional help. The authors have also included some thoughts on how you can evaluate professional help or hospital programs.

Naomi Wolf, *The Beauty Myth* (New York: William Morrow Books, 1991)

Whether you agree or disagree with this author, her book is fascinating and thought provoking. It goes beyond a feminist perspective of weight and society to cover everything from make-up to asceticism to sainthood. This book provides another opportunity to examine external influences on our self-image and our interpretation of physical beauty and its significance in the rest of our lives.

ORGANIZATIONS

Melpomene Institute
1010 University Avenue
St. Paul, MN 55104
(612) 642-1951

**National Association of Anorexia Nervosa and
Associated Disorders (ANAD)**
P.O. Box 7
Highland Park, IL 60035
(708) 831-3438

Anorexia Nervosa and Related Eating Disorders
P.O. Box 5102
Eugene, OR 97405
(503) 344-1144

National Anorexic Aid Society
445 East Granville Road
Worthington, OH 43085
(614) 436-1112

Index

241

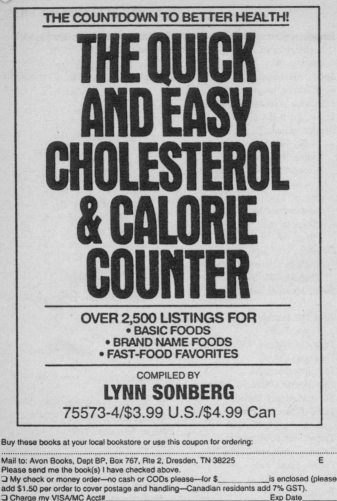